HIDDEN
E P I D E M I C

Silent Oral Infections Cause Most Heart
Attacks and Breast Cancers

HIDDEN
EPIDEMIC

Silent Oral Infections Cause Most Heart
Attacks and Breast Cancers

Thomas E. Levy, MD, JD

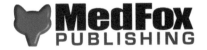

DISCLAIMER

This book is intended to be an information resource only. There is no intent that this book be used for any diagnostic or treatment purposes. A specific physician/patient or dentist/patient relationship is necessary before any medical or dental therapies are initiated. In no manner should this book, or any of the information in this book, be used as a substitute for diagnosis and treatment by a qualified medical and/or dental healthcare professional.

To order additional copies of this book, contact:
MedFox Publishing, LLC
1-866-359-5589
www.MedFoxPub.com
Orders@MedFoxPub.com
2505 Anthem Village Drive, Suite E-582,
Henderson, NV 89052-5529

In memory of my beloved
Mother, Catherine,
who was always my
strongest supporter.

Acknowledgments

To Les and Cindy Nachman, whose support and friendship continue to be invaluable to me in my attempts to get out my medical messages to the world.

To my editor, Dave Nicol, who continues to make my writing so much more intelligible and impactful than it would be otherwise.

To my wife, Lis, and my daughter, Daniela, who motivate me on a daily basis to continue my work.

To Ron Hunninghake, MD, my friend and medical "sounding board" for years now. His perspective always improves mine.

To John Augspurger, DDS, and Corbin Popp, DMD, my friends and dental colleagues, for their consistent help and insights.

And as always, to my friend and mentor, Hal Huggins, DDS, MS for opening my mind and showing me the big picture. I wish he was still here to discuss so very many different things.

Foreword

Our pathway to health and longevity, although a bit daunting, can reward us with a vital and happy life. Staying healthy is a life-long process that requires a certain degree of personal discipline. We must concern ourselves with the food we eat, its source, and how we prepare it. We exercise, drink plenty of water, take our vitamins, and meditate to balance our emotions and spirit. Yet even when we try to do everything possible to maintain our wellness and vitality, we are not granted immunity from the non-communicable chronic diseases like cancer, diabetes, autoimmune disease, hormone imbalance, chronic inflammatory conditions, osteoporosis, heart disease, and early aging that are all around us.

Why?

The human body is an amazing biological system. At the microscopic level, 10% of the cells in our bodies are human and the rest are non-human microorganisms. Functionally, we're an ecosystem that scientists call the microbiome. At the molecular level, we are a massive conglomeration of organic/inorganic chemicals and biomolecules, some stable and some not, that are involved in a free exchange of energy and electrons. A healthy body maintains all of the cells, microorganisms, chemicals, and biomolecules within an organized and balanced system.

However, various factors can disrupt the flow of energy and/or interrupt the balance in the microbiome and throw our bodies into states of chronic disease. This book reveals some of these factors— factors that have been frequently identified by medical researchers yet have failed to be acknowledged by medical and dental practitioners.

In this body of work, Dr. Thomas Levy presents a logical and coherent thesis as to the major cause of this plague that infects a large percentage of the adult population. He presents a powerful case that links the pandemic incidence of chronic degenerative disease to infected teeth, gums, tonsils, cavitations, and sinuses. Most of these infections are insidiously asymptomatic. We don't see or feel them. And even when they do manifest with obvious symptoms, mainstream medicine and dentistry seldom see them as anything more than an isolated condition with no connection to the development of heart disease, cancer, dementia, diabetes, and a host of other chronic degenerative diseases.

To make matters worse, decades of antibiotics overuse have made us more susceptible to an imbalance of our microbiome. When certain pathogenic microorganisms take hold we call it infection. Frequently, these pathogenic microorganisms slide in under the radar. They colonize and set up shop in and around the jaws, teeth, gums and soft tissues of the head and neck. But just because an infection takes up residence in a localized ("focal") area, such as in a tooth, in gum tissue, or in a sinus doesn't mean that its impact is limited to that "focus" of infection.

Contrary to the way we often think, our body does not understand itself as a gathering of isolated parts; rather, it is a unified organism. Pathogens and toxins generated by a "focal" infection can freely circulate throughout the body via our venous and lymphatic systems. We must understand that the effects of these infections are far-reaching and insidious. The medical and dental literature contains copious evidence of these life- and health-threatening effects, and Dr. Levy has exhaustively mined it out and uses it to clearly present his case.

As an integrative biological dentist I face three important challenges on a daily basis. First, I am in a constant battle with infections of the head and neck. Second, I must be able to recognize and properly treat them. Third, and perhaps the most difficult, I must explain the nature of these infections and their implications for overall health and well-being to my patients who think everything's fine. "Hey, when you're symptom-free, pain-free and feeling fine, what could be wrong?" Unfortunately, that's the nature of the silent but deadly oral infections with which we wrestle.

The human body has the amazing capacity to heal, if given the appropriate support. Dr. Levy's informative, well-referenced text provides important information that dramatically exposes the presence and the dangers of silent oral infections. And, not only does he drag these silent destroyers into the light, he gives precise protocols for addressing them. It is priceless information for the clinician and the patient.

In today's world we have many challenges to our health. These challenges come in many forms, but once recognized, understood, and effective therapy is given, the patient can progress toward wellness. As an academic and seeker of truth, I applaud this work. Truth and knowledge brings enlightenment. This work provides all that and more.

Phil Mollica, MS, DMD, NMD
President and Professor
American College of Integrative Medicine and Dentistry

Preface

About 23 years ago I left my practice of adult cardiology. Providentially, I had crossed paths with Dr. Hal Huggins, a dentist with a master's degree in immunology. At the time, and even since in reflection, it appeared to be one of those moments in life for which the saying was first penned: "When the student is ready, the teacher will appear." For many reasons, I was more than ready, and until he appeared, I had no idea where my restlessness in cardiology was going to lead me. It was then that my second medical education was effectively kick-started by this extraordinary person.

Although my traditional training and clinical practice had greatly prepared me to analyze and digest the truth of what I was about to learn, the education Dr. Huggins provided was far more substantial. Sadly, the vast majority of what he taught and frequently demonstrated to me remains unknown or actively disparaged by both mainstream medicine and mainstream dentistry.

Being perhaps more open-minded than intellectual, I simply observed what Dr. Huggins was doing in performing the Total Dental Revisions on his patients, along with the clinical and laboratory results he was achieving.

After mercury and infected teeth or infected implants were properly removed, I saw abnormal blood tests normalize or dramatically improve. I watched patients with advanced chronic degenerative diseases, including multiple sclerosis, Alzheimer's, Parkinson's, and even ALS make substantial improvement during the couple of weeks they spent at the clinic.

These were improvements that I was trained to believe were simply not possible in any of these diseases — ever.

A few multiple sclerosis patients actually took their first steps after being in a wheelchair for years after completing the program. Some individuals with dramatically elevated antinuclear antibody levels seen in lupus and other autoimmune diseases would no longer have detectable levels at the end of their visit. Others would have similar results within a month or two on follow-up blood testing.

Repeat blood testing in gout patients who had extremely elevated uric levels for years would demonstrate normalized levels. These and many other incredible, dramatically positive health responses were common. Intellectual honesty would not allow me to deny what was happening before my very eyes. I was compelled to start working with Dr. Huggins and learn everything I could from him.

During the time I spent studying with Dr. Huggins, I learned of the toxicity of the mercury in all the "silver" fillings put in so many people for so many years. I witnessed the enormous toxicity inflicted by many root canal-treated teeth, along with other infected teeth. I repeatedly witnessed the extremely common finding of infected cavitations at old extraction sites, something that remains largely unknown to "modern" dentistry. And I witnessed the incredible therapeutic power of intravenous vitamin C, something that is not even mentioned in the most current of medical textbooks.

An extraordinary mentor, and one of the best friends I have ever had, Dr. Huggins passed away November 29, 2014. I will always miss him immensely, especially as I later "discovered" new ideas that I knew he would so passionately love analyzing and discussing.

Twenty-three years after we first met, and 10 books later (one coauthored with Dr. Huggins), I'm still working to disseminate his enormous body of work, and even occasionally to perhaps expand upon it. To this day, there is nothing he ever told me that has proven to be scientifically wrong.

One of the most important things I learned is that an infected tooth can destroy a person's health very rapidly. The toxicity of the infection in a root canal-canal treated tooth was always at the top of the list as a factor that would ultimately compromise health, both as a cause of chronic disease as well as a primary reason why such disease continued to evolve and worsen. Two of my books, coauthored with Robert Kulacz, DDS (*The Roots of Disease* in 2002 and *The Toxic Tooth* in 2014) addressed this toxicity of root canal-treated teeth in great detail by examining the pathophysiology and the pertinent scientific articles.

After the release of *The Toxic Tooth*, I felt that Dr. Kulacz and I had presented a very definitive evaluation and assessment of the scientific truth about root canals and their involvement in chronic degenerative diseases. We especially emphasized the cause-and-effect relationship between the pathogens in root canals and the formation of the blood clots that result in most heart attacks. The information in that book is as valid today as it was when we were writing it. However, medicine and science evolve, understandings improve and become more comprehensive, and the clinical practices of both dentistry and medicine must evolve as well. That is what all patients expect and deserve.

Early in 2016, while accompanying a close friend to the dentist to have several root canal-treated teeth extracted, a 3D cone beam imaging study of her teeth was performed to best define the pathology that was present and to optimize the subsequent treatment plan for the extractions. There were three root canal-treated teeth in a row in the upper left maxilla. However, the adjacent molar showed a huge radiolucency, or dark space, (chronic apical periodontitis, or CAP) around each root tip. Furthermore, the bony floor of the sinus had eroded away completely where it had been in contact with the roots of this tooth. There was a large fluid level in the sinus, as my friend had been suffering with chronic sinusitis for many years.

I asked a simple question of my friend: "Do you have any pain at all on that side of the mouth, and does it ever hurt when you chew?" The answer was simple and definitive: "No."

Radiologically, the infected tooth looked like it was acutely abscessed. However, this was obviously not the case, since it was pain-free, and it was performing its mechanical function of chewing without any problem at all. Instead, this was a severely infected tooth that had never received a dental procedure, and yet it was completely asymptomatic. Intuitively, I absolutely knew that the toxicity of this tooth had to be as bad or even worse than the adjacent root canals. They had not eroded into the sinus, but this tooth had. I reluctantly informed my friend that she needed to have an additional extraction, since her primary concern was to optimize her long-term health.

This finding both fascinated me and upset me. How many people like my friend have silent yet severely infected teeth? If this was a common occurrence, then the main reason for most heart attacks (to which root canals already were demonstrated to have a cause-and-effect relationship) and breast cancers was being routinely overlooked, or perhaps more accurately, never discovered.

As it turns out, my initial research in PubMed revealed that CAP is extremely common, especially with root canal-treated teeth, but also quite often on untreated teeth. The literature also showed that CAP was reliably **_more_** toxic than many root canal-treated teeth without significant CAP.

Additionally, the literature conclusively demonstrated that regular dental X-rays often miss teeth with significant CAP (see Appendix D to see how effectively CAP can "hide" on a regular dental X-ray). However, the 3D cone beam imaging technology reliably reveals all CAP teeth except when the degree of CAP is very minimal.

The studies that demonstrate the pandemic prevalence of CAP in the general population along with the large volume of medical literature linking periodontitis with a host of degenerative diseases, brought me to a startling conclusion. One of the main reasons for the majority of deaths from diseases like heart disease and cancer in the United States and around the world were due to the toxicity and disseminated pathogens from asymptomatic infected teeth! These "hidden killers" are seldom discovered and they are rarely extracted properly or otherwise effectively treated when they are found by accident.

This reality also explains why so many cancer patients initially experience positive responses to various treatments but later have recurrences or even new cancers. And why heart disease continues to evolve after angioplasties and bypasses, as would certainly be expected if the dental infections feeding the coronary artery inflammation are never identified and addressed.

For these reasons, then, *Hidden Epidemic* has been written. I affectionately call my friend "Patient Zero" in helping to reveal what is arguably the largest, most chronic, and most deadly epidemic to attack longevity and health in history. Review the data, decide for yourself, and then decide whether you need to obtain 3D cone beam imaging of your mouth before your chest pain or breast lump appears.

— Thomas E. Levy, MD, JD

Table of Contents

PART ONE: Undeniable Evidence

PART TWO: Underlying Empirical Science

Chapter 4 - 75

Increased Oxidative Stress:
The Common Cause of All Diseases

PART FOUR: Diagnosis and Treatment

PART FIVE: More Help

Introduction

Collectively, heart disease and cancer account for more deaths in the developed world than all of the other chronic degenerative diseases put together. Add to this the amount of suffering that is endured prior to death, especially in the case of cancer, and it is apparent that the public health as well as the massive financial impact of these two disease categories is overwhelmingly great.

To the great detriment of a patient's well-being in particular and society as a whole, modern medicine primarily addresses the pharmaceutical alleviation of disease-associated symptoms. For a patient in intense pain, pain relief is primary. Medical treatment may go a little beyond the pain to remediate additional symptoms, but rarely is the etiology of a given disease determined and eradicated. As a consequence, a full resolution of the disease is seldom realized.

Similarly, modern dentistry, first and foremost, seeks to address the symptom of pain. If the pain in an infected tooth can be relieved, it is largely assumed by most dentists that the optimal treatment for that tooth has been rendered. Modern dentistry makes no systematic effort to identify how the dental infections it treats every day impact a patient's general health.

By their very nature, however, most of the disease-causing infections mentioned in this book are asymptomatic—without pain. So it is vitally important that medical practitioners, dentists, and especially patients come to this stark realization:

A lack of symptoms, especially pain, is not equivalent to freedom from disease-causing infection and its ultimate devastation.

Even a superficial review of the pertinent medical literature reveals that dental infections (mostly free from pain) greatly impact the general health of the population. That review also shows that there is nothing else that even remotely generates as profound a negative health impact. Nevertheless, there is little to no ongoing exchange of information between most dentists and physicians, much to the detriment of the patients being treated.

For centuries, the concept of asymptomatic focal infections as a basis for degenerative disease has been a topic of debate. It has been studied, discussed, and now ***demonstrated*** ***conclusively*** that these infections can persist in the body for years and that they can and do exert a continuous and substantial negative impact on the health of a patient.

Yet, mainstream medicine and mainstream dentistry both continue to largely dismiss any suggestion of a connection of chronic degenerative disease to focal infection. Hence they see no practical application of this concept in the day-to-day treatment of patients with any of these diseases. Indeed, most modern practitioners of medicine and dentistry remain completely unaware of, or at least very unfamiliar with, the large body of scientific literature indicating focal infection to be the cause and aggravator of a wide variety of chronic medical conditions.

The emergence of sophisticated diagnostic technology, especially 3D cone beam imaging of the teeth, has revealed many significant focal infections that were never even suspected to be present in the past. The vast majority of the adult population of the world has at least one significant tooth infection. Yet, these teeth nearly always go undiscovered and are rarely addressed. Nevertheless, it is these teeth, along with infected tonsils and infected gums that *cause the vast majority of heart attacks and cases of breast cancer.*

Furthermore, rarely do heart disease and cancer resolve in a definitive way when these dental infections remain unidentified and unaddressed. Usually the best that optimal traditional medical care affords such situations is a stabilization of the condition. However, and this cannot be overemphasized, when dental focal infections are definitely remedied, heart disease and even advanced cancers have a real opportunity of substantial resolution and even cure by all measurable standards...and not just rarely. When the disease is not extremely advanced, such disease resolution will be the rule, not the exception. However, until searching for and eradicating such focal infections becomes routine, the statistical chance of complete disease resolution will be minimized.

The prevalence of this hidden epidemic of disease-causing infections of the oral cavity is more devastating than any other disease or epidemic that has ever plagued mankind. There is undeniable evidence that asymptomatic oral infections reside in the majority of the adult population. The incidence of the chronic degenerative diseases and the massive financial burden they create for individuals and all of society is enormous and unsustainable. Medical journals are teeming with evidence of demonstrable links between these infections and heart disease, cancer, neurological disease, vascular diseases, and increased all-cause mortality.

Modern imaging equipment (such as 3D cone beam imaging) and simple blood tests (such as for C-reactive protein) provide reliable ways to detect asymptomatic oral infections and to monitor remediation efforts. Armed with the information in *The Hidden Epidemic* and these powerful detection and monitoring tools, patients, dentists, and medical practitioners can begin the important work of identifying and eliminating this arch-enemy to physical and financial health. May it be so!

The Prevalence of Undetected, Silent Oral Infections

Overview

The teeth, gums, jawbone cavitations, tonsils, and sinuses are the primary sites of oral infection in humans. All of these sites facilitate the existence of pathogenic pools that are generally chronic and painless, proliferating quietly under the radar. They reliably dispense pathogens and toxins throughout the body via the circulatory and lymphatic systems "24/7," frequently initiating seemingly unrelated biological havoc at one or more distant sites. Even though the prevalence of these infections reaches *beyond* epidemic proportions, they receive little attention because of their invisible status.

Certainly, if these infections in the mouth, throat, and sinuses were of minor consequence, there would be little reason for further discussion. But, as this book will clearly demonstrate, that is simply not the case.

This chapter presents and discusses statistics from many published research studies that indicate how frequently these insidious infections occur. The staggering life and resource costs that chronic degenerative diseases impose on society are discussed in Chapter 2. Chapter 3 then exposes the startling data from the peer-reviewed medical literature that demonstrate the undeniable link, and very arguably, the cause-and-effect relationship between oral infections and many of those same chronic degenerative diseases.

Almost by definition, asymptomatic infections will remain undiagnosed since there are no symptoms to pressure a diagnosis.

Almost by definition, asymptomatic infections will remain undiagnosed since there are no symptoms to pressure a diagnosis. Therefore, obtaining verifiable statistics presents some real challenges. However, developing highly predictive data using logical extrapolation can nevertheless reveal the scope of the underlying problem. For example, if studies suggest that over 95% of root canal-treated teeth harbor infection, and that 35% of adults have at least one such tooth, it is reasonable to assume that a minimum of nearly 33% (one in three) adults in the general population have an asymptomatic dental infection based on that evidence alone. However, the problem is even worse and more widespread.

The sheer number of these infections is alarming, but if, as the research indicates, these infections cause and worsen cancer, heart disease, dementia, and most other chronic degenerative diseases, we are in the midst of a "modern plague" that surpasses any pandemic ever seen. And we also have the opportunity to reverse a great deal of disease never before considered reversible.

Below, you will find a careful presentation and discussion regarding two very common sources of oral infection (root canal-treated teeth and chronic apical periodontitis) and their frequency of occurrence. The prevalence of these two infections by themselves adequately demonstrates the epidemic nature of asymptomatic oral infections without even considering the other dental, periodontal, and tonsillar sources of oral infections, all of which provoke even more chronic disease throughout the body.

...literally 100% of 5,000 examined root canal-treated teeth were infected.

Root Canal-Treated Teeth

The root canal procedure, one of the most performed dental treatments of our time, is responsible for the most common chronic oral cavity infection. While some would argue that most root canal-treated tooth are infection-free, recent data showed that literally 100% of 5,000 examined root canal-treated teeth were infected.[1] That means that those who have one or more root canal-treated teeth can reliably assume that they have a chronic oral infection. Although all such infected teeth are not of equal negative clinical impact, it is still important to realize that none of them are completely free of pathogens and toxins.

Depending on your information source, somewhere between 15 and 25 million root canal procedures are performed annually in the United States. But regardless of the precise number, the growth of this procedure remains steady and substantial. In Denmark, for example, the annual number of root canal procedures increased by over 30% between 1977 and 2003, from 268,223 to 364,867.[2] It remains an enormously popular and common

Table 1-1 Prevalence of Root Canal-Treated Teeth in Various Countries

Country	Total Teeth	% Root Canal-Treated Teeth
Kosovar[3]	4,131	2.3%
Croatia[4]		8.5%
Italy[5]	9,423	11.4%
Belgium[6]	11,117	12.2%
Serbia[7]	3,526	12.5%
Latvia[8]	7,065	18.0%
Japan[9]	16,232	21.0%
Brazil[10]	29,467	21.4%

procedure around the world, and it appears that the number of these procedures is only continuing to increase. Consider the statistical findings in the studies presented in Table 1-1.

Admittedly, the statistical variance of root canal-filled teeth in these studies is substantial. Much of this variance is likely related to the financial ability of various populations to pay for endodontic care. Even at the lowest rate, however, 2.3% of all teeth is a significant number of teeth. On the other hand, 21.4% (an average of 5 to 6 teeth per mouth) is astronomical. Considering recent findings that all root canal-treated teeth are still chronically infected, this number is particularly frightening.

Many studies suggest that at least 50% of patients have at least one root canal and in some patient subsets, the percentage is substantially higher. With regard to public health impact, these statistics are even more disturbing. Consider the information in Table 1-2.

Although similar studies for the United States were not found, the American Association of

Table 1-2 Prevalence of Root Canal-Treated Teeth per Person

Country	Number of Adults	% with Root Canals
Brazil[10]	1,401	47.6%
Croatia[11]	135	59.0%
Italy[12]	672	87.0%

Endodontists estimates that 22.3 million root canal procedures were performed in 2006.[13] According to the U.S. Census Bureau, there were 219.8 million adults in the U.S. in that same year.[14] It is safe to assume, then, that approximately 10% of American adults were subjected to this procedure during that one-year period. And even if the incidence of this procedure has remained static, it is reasonable to assume that a majority of the adults in the United States has at least one root canal-treated tooth.

The American Association of Endodontists estimates that 22.3 million root canal procedures were performed in 2006.

Even though toxicity has a quantitative as well as a qualitative aspect, just one root canal-treated tooth can profoundly and negatively impact heart and general health. This is especially true when there is X-ray evidence of chronic apical periodontitis (CAP) as well, which is very often the case. Certain teeth are especially susceptible, with a CAP prevalence of 86% in root canal-treated maxillary molars noted in a French population.[15]

Chronic Apical Periodontitis

Periodontitis is an inflammation due to infection in the tissues around the teeth (gums). Chronic apical periodontitis (CAP) is a common, often long-standing infection residing around or along the tip (apex) of a tooth. CAP is also called periapical periodontitis, or periradicular periodontitis.

CAP shares the following characteristics with general periodontal disease:[16]

1. Both are chronic oral cavity infections.
2. CAP is the most advanced form of periodontitis and often evolves over time from lesser degrees of periodontitis.
3. The pathogen profile of each is virtually identical.
4. Both result in the elevation of inflammatory biomarkers reflective of body-wide increases in oxidative stress.

CAP, as an ***advanced*** form of general periodontitis, must be linked to all of the diseases to which the ***lesser*** infection of general periodontitis has already been linked. It is of great importance to understand and realize that CAP in its ***painless, silent form*** is an extremely common finding in the general population. However, CAP teeth always contain similar pathogen profiles, whether asymptomatic or causing pain.[17] This includes CAP in ***both*** root canal-treated teeth and in untreated teeth. And when something is painless and asymptomatic, discoverable only by X-ray, it will never be known to the physician unless incidentally found in the workup and treatment of other symptomatic teeth by the dentist, and the dentist makes the effort to let the physician know of the CAP presence.

Table 1-3 Prevalence of Chronic Apical Periodontitis in Various Countries

Country	Total Patients	Total Teeth	% CAP	% CAP in Root Canal-Treated Teeth
Turkey[20]	1,000	24,433	0.8%*	18.0%
Ireland[21]	302	7,427	1.6%*	25.0%
Spain[22]	180	4,453	2.9%*	65.0%
Belgium[23]		4,617	6.6%†	40.0%
Portugal[24]	179		27.0%†	22.0%
France[25]	344	7,555	1.7%*	32.0%
Manhattan (USA)[26]			5.1%†	38.0%
Holland[27]	184		5.2%*	39.0%
Sweden[28]			3.3%*	13.9%
Sweden[28]			6.8%*	17.7%
Norway[29]			3.5%†	44.0%
Turkey[30]	242		n/a	46.0%
Brazil[31]			3.4%†	51.4%
India[32]	1,340	30,098	4.3%*	37.0%
Iran[33]		1,064	n/a	52.0%
Finland[34]			9.0%*	39.0%
Nigeria[35]		All teeth examined: 74.0%		
Saudi Arabia[36]		234	n/a	59.0%
Palestine[37]			8.3%*	

* % CAP in All Teeth   † % CAP in Untreated Teeth

The negative body-wide impact that periodontitis has been established to have on general health, along with its cause-and-effect impact on heart disease and its strong correlation with so many other diseases, should make periodontitis a public health issue of great concern. Furthermore, the high prevalence of the most advanced form of periodontitis (CAP) on dental X-rays should ramp up this concern even higher. CAP develops as a result of an infected, necrotic pulp in an untreated tooth or as a result of failed or poorly-performed endodontic treatment.[18] So, regardless of whether CAP appears on an untreated tooth or is the unsuccessful outcome of a root canal treatment, it is an infected, highly toxic condition that must be properly addressed to best safeguard the health of the patient.

Many studies have examined the prevalence of CAP in different populations. In a group of Spanish adults, a very high prevalence of CAP was reported in both untreated and in root canal-treated teeth. At least one tooth with CAP was discovered in 41% of non-smoking patients and 74% of the smoking patients.[19] This is a very significant statistic as one chronically infected tooth is capable of promoting any of a number of diseases or even directly causing a heart attack. The prevalence of CAP in other populations has been examined in many studies. See some of those results in Table 1-3.

The primary point of all of the statistics on CAP just cited above is straightforward: CAP, while variably present in different populations, is nevertheless very common, typically discovered incidentally and presenting in a painless, asymptomatic state.

Conclusion

Silent oral infections are extremely common, based just on the prevalence of root canal-treated teeth and chronic apical periodontitis. With these two hotspots alone, it is very likely that a substantial majority of adults are playing host to at least one of these focal infections. When other types of oral infections are included, that percentage only increases.

Many dentists and doctors will state that oral infections are not nearly as prevalent as the statistics above indicate. Others claim the theory that a focal infection can cause disease in other parts of the body has been disproven. Still others argue that these oral infections are not significantly consequential. Rarely do these naysayers present scientific evidence to support their arguments, and when they do, it's usually only one or two studies that have been conducted by the very groups that have a vested interest in the outcome.

Before you make up your mind, take the time to read and consider the evidence presented in the next two chapters...

The Pandemic Incidence of Chronic Degenerative Diseases

Overview

Chapter 1 showed the widespread, nearly ubiquitous, prevalence of asymptomatic oral infections. As part of the justification for the need to address these infections, this chapter will discuss the simultaneous and pandemic incidence of chronic degenerative diseases.

Some might argue that the fact the two events are concurrent does not prove that one causes the other. That is true, but if there is a demonstrable, likely causal link between the asymptomatic oral infections and chronic degenerative diseases, as the data presented in Chapter 3 clearly demonstrates, the following statistics are both cause for alarm and a reason for hope.

The worldwide treatment of chronic degenerative diseases costs trillions of dollars annually. If there is even a possibility that oral infections are the source of the toxins and pathogens that cause most of these chronic diseases, an unprecedented opportunity for effective disease treatment and prevention waits. Unlike the lifelong symptomatic medical treatment of chronic diseases, these oral infections can be completely resolved in a straightforward, relatively painless, and exponentially less expensive manner.

Cumulatively, the four most prevalent chronic degenerative diseases are cancer, cardiovascular/heart disease, diabetes, and dementia. These conditions are probably the most dreaded and certainly the most expensive in every measurable way. Individually, nationally, and globally, there is more than sufficient reason to consider the potential savings, on all levels, of preventing, resolving, and even curing these diseases.

Based on numbers published on The National Cancer Institute website, cancer will claim over 500,000 American lives this year.

Cancer

Statistics regarding cancer prevalence and costs can be dizzying, to say the least. Global costs for treatment approaches one **_trillion_** dollars.[1] Expected new cases in the U.S. per year and annual deaths are in the hundreds of thousands.

Based on numbers published on The National Cancer Institute website, cancer will claim over

500,000 American lives this year. Over 1.6 million new cases will be diagnosed this year. And annual cancer treatment costs, not counting associated non-treatment costs, will fall between $130 and $150 billion.[2]

A group of researchers analyzed the aggregate costs for five of the major forms of cancer in the United States. Here's a summary of their projections for 2020 for the three most expensive types of cancer:[3]

> *...your chances of being diagnosed with cancer in your lifetime are 2 out of 5.*

- **Breast Cancer**
  - Initial treatment: $6.85 Billion
  - Continuing care: $8.9 Billion
  - Last year of care: $4.75 Billion
- **Colorectal Cancer**
  - Initial treatment: $7.23 Billion
  - Continuing care: $4.91 Billion
  - Last year of care: $5.27 Billion
- **Prostate Cancer**
  - Initial treatment: $6.02 Billion
  - Continuing care: $8.81 Billion
  - Last year of care: $1.52 Billion

To help put this all in perspective, it may be helpful to look at the costs in more personal terms. For example, your chances of being diagnosed with cancer in your lifetime are 2 out of 5. The average cost of cancer surgery, depending on the type of cancer, ranges from $30,000 to $56,000. Chemotherapy can cost from nearly $70,000 to over $100,000 for **_12 months_** of care. Radiation treatments for 3 months will cost over $35,000. Plus, there are additional hidden costs of gas, parking, lodging, meals away from home, childcare, nutritional supplements, special equipment, special clothing, and other "incidentals." Although survival rates vary by cancer type, currently the overall odds of "cancer survival," usually couched in terms of living 5 additional years, are about 3 in 5. In other words, you will likely spend well over $200,000 to treat your cancer, endure the unpleasant side effects, be unable to work, and still have a 2 in 5 chance of losing the battle.

> *Ultimately, the huge cost of national cancer treatment will be extracted from those who pay taxes and insurance premiums.*

Even if you and everyone in your home dodge the cancer bullet, the reality is that you're still going to pay. Yes, the government and insurance companies pay the biggest share of the bill. But, both pass along **_ALL_** these costs, plus substantial administrative fees, to taxpayers and insurance policy holders. Ultimately, the huge cost of national cancer treatment will be extracted from those who pay taxes and insurance premiums.

Cardiovascular Disease and Heart Disease

The prevalence of cardiovascular/heart disease (including coronary heart disease and stroke) for Americans without diabetes is about 16% or about one in six. That number increases to about 68%, or two out of three, for those who have diabetes.[4]

...the cost of treating cardiovascular disease ...will exceed $1 trillion by 2035.

According to the Centers for Disease Control, one in four deaths in the U.S. are caused by heart disease. Each year, about 610,000 people die from it and on average an American dies with a heart attack every minute.[5] The American Heart Association reported that the cost of treating cardiovascular disease in 2015, including medical and indirect costs, was about $555 billion. They predict those costs will exceed ***$1 trillion*** by 2035.[6]

Diabetes

According to the American Diabetes Association (ADA), about 29.1 million Americans (9.3%) have diabetes. For seniors the prevalence soars to about 25.9%. Diabetes is the 7th leading cause of death in the United States. In addition, there are several other conditions that are considered to be complications of diabetes including hypertension (high blood pressure), dyslipidemia (high low-density cholesterol and elevated triglycerides), death from cardiovascular disease, heart attack, stroke, blindness, and vitamin C disease, and amputations.[7]

Diabetes is the 7th leading cause of death in the United States.

The medical costs associated with the treatment of diabetes exceed $245 billion per year for those actually diagnosed with diabetes. The ADA estimates that 8 million cases are undiagnosed.[7] The incidence of diabetes is expected to quadruple by 2050.[8,9] Even with no rise in current per case treatment costs, the total costs would exceed ***$1 trillion***.

Dementia

The Alzheimer's Association reports that Alzheimer's is the 6th leading cause of death in the United States and that more than 5 million individuals are currently living with it. Researchers predict that as the population in the U.S. ages, the incidence of dementia will increase dramatically. They also say that in 2017 the nation will spend $259 million treating all dementias, and by 2050 that price tag is expected to top ***$1.1 trillion***.[10]

It bears repeating that the government and insurance companies can only reimburse medical providers from taxes and premiums. The citizens will bear the costs.

Conclusion

The financial costs of treating the four diseases discussed above are about $1 trillion per year in the United States. According to Forbes, 45.3% of the 131 million American households pay taxes,[11] but most of those do not pay insurance premiums as well. That means 59 million households will bear the annual cost of these four diseases, or about $16,700 per household. And, these costs are far from static. They are rising exponentially faster than most other goods, services, and wages in our economy. By 2050 total treatment costs could be as high as **_$4 trillion per year_**. These costs are unsustainable.

> *That means $59 million households will bear the annual cost of these four diseases, or about $16,700 per household. And, these costs are far from static.*

And in addition to the financial burden, there are the incalculable costs of personal physical/emotional suffering, the stress on families, and the toll on national productivity.

As will be demonstrated in Chapter 3, the vast majority of significant chronic degenerative diseases has been linked to asymptomatic oral infections. It is quite probable, as the evidence presented in the next chapter demonstrates, that many of these diseases could be prevented, resolved and/or cured by clearing up the focal infections that cause and support them. Therefore, early detection, early diagnosis, and the effective treatment of asymptomatic oral infections should be a personal and even a national priority.

The Demonstrable Link Between Oral Infections and Chronic Diseases

Overview

A very large number of scientific studies link gum infections (periodontitis) to an alarming host of different diseases and medical conditions.[1] However, with the exception of coronary heart disease which has a demonstrable ***cause-and-effect*** connection to periodontal pathogens, the vast majority of these studies only examine the statistical correlation between these maladies and general periodontitis. General periodontitis is the most easily diagnosed and the least severe of periodontal infections. Relatively few studies have investigated disease connections between the ***most advanced*** and ***most toxic*** of periodontal infections, namely, chronic apical periodontitis (CAP).

Therefore, ***at the very least***, any disease or medical condition that can be attributed to or strongly linked to general periodontitis will be as much or more connected to any tooth with CAP. Even though the list of medical conditions below provides an overview of the enormous negative clinical impact of general periodontitis, all of the conditions **_can_ _also_ _reliably_ _be_ _correlated_ _to_ _an_ _asymptomatic_ _CAP_ _tooth_** as well, with or without root canal treatment.

> *...all of the conditions can also reliably be correlated to an asymptomatic CAP tooth... with or without root canal treatment.*

Such periodontitis-disease connections with documentation in the scientific literature include the following:

✓ Heart disease
✓ Cancer
✓ Alzheimer's disease and other neurological/psychiatric diseases
✓ All-cause mortality
✓ Abnormal calcification in blood vessels and heart
✓ Anemia of chronic disease
✓ Arthritis, especially rheumatoid
✓ Body-wide increased oxidative stress biomarkers
✓ Cerebrovascular disease
✓ Diabetes
✓ Erectile dysfunction
✓ HIV infection
✓ Hypertension (high blood pressure)

- ✓ Inflammatory bowel disease
- ✓ Metabolic syndrome
- ✓ Osteoporosis
- ✓ Osteonecrosis of the jawbone
- ✓ Preeclampsia, maternal hypertension, maternal anemia, low birth weight, preterm birth
- ✓ Prostatitis and elevated levels of prostate-specific antigen (PSA)
- ✓ Pulmonary disease
- ✓ Sudden hearing loss
- ✓ Systemic lupus erythematosus
- ✓ Vascular disease

Periodontitis in all forms, and especially in its most advanced CAP form, is clearly responsible for causing systemic, body-wide disease in addition to the universally recognized localized infections in the gums, jawbone, and tooth socket. Even though it originates in the mouth, periodontitis is just as much (or more) a general disease of the body as diabetes. The laundry list of medical conditions linked to periodontitis as itemized above, along with the well-established and strong link between periodontitis and increased all-cause mortality, establishes this reality beyond all doubt.

Each of the following subsections will demonstrate some of these associations with specific diseases and medical conditions.

Periodontitis and Heart Disease

The large body of scientific literature documenting the connection between periodontal disease and heart disease establishes that periodontal disease is not only a risk factor for coronary heart disease, but that it increases that risk independently from the other known risk factors.[2-10]

Root canal-treated teeth have now been proven to have a direct cause-and-effect relationship with... myocardial infarctions.

Root canal-treated teeth have now been proven to have a direct ***cause-and-effect*** relationship with the formation of the blood clots that acutely block off the blood flow in the coronary arteries and cause myocardial infarctions. In 78% of 101 patients presenting with myocardial infarctions and occluded coronary arteries, the DNA of pathogens typical for infections in root canal-treated teeth was found in the occluding blood clots after they were aspirated out of the coronary arteries via angiographic access. The testing for this DNA utilized the sensitive and sophisticated polymerase chain reaction (PCR) technology. The pathogens typical for periodontal (gum) disease, which usually seed the pathogens that infect the tooth pulp prior to receiving a root canal treatment, were found in 35%

of this patient group. Furthermore, the concentration of the pathogen-related DNA in these blood clots was **16 times (1,600%) higher** than in the surrounding arterial blood.[11]

This is the "smoking-gun" study: **_Root canal-treated teeth are the direct cause for the vast majority of heart attacks, period_**.

> Root canal-treated teeth are the direct cause for the vast majority of heart attacks, period.

An examination of the scientific literature published prior to the study above had already shown that oral pathogens are consistently present in coronary atherosclerotic plaques and are likely the entire reason why coronary arteries develop the chronic inflammation seen at the outset of all coronary artery disease. Multiple investigators have found the DNA of the pathogens typically associated with oral infections in coronary and carotid artery atheromas.[12-14] Another group that examined tissue specimens from 38 coronary heart disease patients after atherectomies (plaque removal via catheter) found bacterial DNA in **_all_** of the specimens, with an overall diversity in excess of 50 different species. Fungal DNA was found in 92% (35 of 38) of those patients.[15] Furthermore, control specimens taken postmortem from normal coronary arteries did not contain any bacterial DNA.[16] Another study found that not only did there appear to be a specific immune response associated with atherosclerosis, but that the presence of periodontal pathogens appeared to enhance the **maintenance** of the inflammatory immune response.[17]

Another study that utilized PCR testing to detect the presence of bacterial DNA strongly supports a cause-and-effect relationship between oral pathogens from root canal-treated teeth and periodontal disease with coronary atherosclerosis. Pericardial fluid specimens from coronary heart disease patients obtained post-mortem were examined. A sizeable majority of these patients had oral pathogen-related DNA detected in the pericardial fluid specimens. Furthermore, the more advanced the coronary disease had been while the patient was alive, the greater the total amount of bacterial DNA was found in the fluid.[18]

... the DNA from pathogens typical for root canal-treated teeth were found in a majority of ruptured intracranial aneurysms.

Consistent with the seeding of coronary atheromas with oral pathogens of root canal and periodontal origin, it would appear that the same process takes place in some cerebrovascular arteries. By PCR testing, the DNA from pathogens typical for root canal-treated teeth were found in a majority of ruptured intracranial aneurysms. The specimens were gathered predominately from

aneurysm clipping operations, with some specimens obtained at autopsy.[19] Perhaps a long enough
exposure to oral pathogens weakens the cerebrovascular artery and causes the aneurysms to form
in the first place and eventually to rupture. Another
possibility is that the abnormal blood flow patterns
around pre-existing aneurysms could make them
more likely areas to permit bacterial seeding to take
place and further weaken the vessel wall.

The cause-and-effect relationship between
root canal-treated teeth and the formation of blood
clots causing heart attacks published by Pessi
et al. described above is further supported by a
large statistical study.[20] This study examined the
correlation between the presence of root canal-
treated teeth and the presence of coronary heart
disease. It showed that "...those with a greater
self-reported history of EF [root canal treatments]
were more likely to have CHD [coronary heart
disease] than those reporting no history of EF." A
similar conclusion was reported by a second group
of researchers.[21] Both studies reached the same
conclusion, namely: ***If you have one or more root
canal-treated teeth, you have an increased chance
of heart attack.***

While an untreated tooth with CAP will often
promote atherosclerosis even more than an infected
tooth that has been given an optimally-performed
root canal treatment, this does not remove the
risk of heart attack as effectively as the proper

extraction of that tooth. In the informed consent for receiving a root canal treatment, this information must be communicated to the patient. The informed patient can then weigh the pros and cons of the procedure and decide if it is their best option. Certainly, many patients will still not want a tooth extraction; they just need to have all of the information before deciding on a root canal procedure, or even perhaps before deciding on an extraction to be followed by an immediate dental implant, a sequence proving to be a very effective and non-toxic alternative to tooth extraction alone. More than anything else, most patients simply do not want to deal with a missing tooth.

Ironically, cardiologists and internists alike now agree that inflammation of the lining (endothelial cell layer) of the coronary artery is the primary cause for initiating and evolving the atherosclerotic plaques.[22] Furthermore, it is generally agreed that this causative inflammation is chronic in nature.[23] However, inflammation always results from increased oxidative stress, and that increased oxidative stress always results directly from toxins, other pro-oxidants, and reactive oxygen species. So what usually causes the increased oxidative stress inside the coronary arteries of chronic heart disease patients?

The most common reason for ongoing chronic inflammation in the body is due to the increased oxidative stress generated by a ***chronic infection*** *or pathogen colonization*, as has been documented to be present in all or practically all diseased coronary arteries. However, in spite of this established presence of oral pathogen DNA at all stages of atherosclerosis, the consistent conclusion of too many heart attack-treating doctors is that their patients really just had bad luck. While having a chronically inflamed coronary artery would never be associated with good luck, there is a consistent reason for its presence: focal arterial infection with its associated toxicity and chronic inflammation. And this almost always comes from chronically infected teeth—most often root canal-treated, and/or from chronic periodontitis. Every biological event occurs for a reason, even if it is not commonly known or appreciated.

> *Some of these studies reported as much as a 2.5-fold increase in some cancers associated with advanced periodontitis.*

Periodontitis and Cancer

Many studies have linked the incidence of a myriad of cancers with periodontal disease. Some of these studies reported as much as a 2.5-fold increase in some cancers associated with advanced periodontitis.[24-30] A sampling of specific types of cancer that have been associated with periodontitis follows.

Pancreatic Cancer

A review of the medical literature addressing patients with a history of periodontal disease found a positive association between these oral infections and increased pancreatic cancer risk.[31] At least two large studies, one with 50,000 professional males aged 40-75 years over a 16-year period,[32] and another with over 200,000 subjects,[33] also found links between periodontitis and pancreatic cancer risk. The larger study also found independent links between periodontal disease and other medical conditions and diseases, including diabetes, hyperlipidemia, allergies, viral hepatitis, peptic ulcer, pancreatitis, and diseases associated with smoking and alcohol use.

> There is also evidence now that microbes like Fusobacterium [a significant periodontal pathogen], are "significantly enriched in breast tissue from women with malignant disease."

Breast Cancer

There is also evidence now that microbes like *Fusobacterium* **[a significant periodontal pathogen]**, are "significantly enriched in breast tissue from women with malignant disease."[34] This fits perfectly with the concept that the lymphatics draining infected teeth and gums and extending down into the breasts allow a steady suffusion of oral pathogens and their related toxins, keeping much of the breast tissue in a continued state of increased oxidative stress. As will be discussed later, increased oxidative stress is **_always paramount_** in setting the stage for malignant transformation.

Colon Cancer

Fusobacterium, which was just discussed as it relates to breast cancer, has already been strongly linked to colon cancer.[35] It has been proposed that this common oral pathogen might act to further promote carcinogenesis due to secreted factors that further promote a pro-inflammatory microenvironment.[36] Without any stretch of the imagination it also follows that infected gums can be a ready source for this pathogen to seed the gut and colon simply via swallowing.[37]

> *Fusobacterium... has already been strongly linked to colon cancer.*

Head, Neck, Oral Cavity, Esophageal Cancers

A host of researchers have found significant associations between periodontitis and cancers of the oral cavity, including the tongue.[38-45] Several other studies demonstrated a link between periodontal disease and carcinogenesis of the head and neck region.[46-48] It is important to note that several of these studies tie the genesis of these cancers to pathogens commonly seen in periodontal disease.

The researchers concluded that subjects with periodontal disease are at a significantly increased risk of developing lung cancer.

Lung Cancer

In 2016, researchers performed a statistical analysis of several previously published studies to identify an observable link between periodontitis and lung cancer. The analyzed studies had a combined cohort of 321,420 subjects. The researchers concluded that subjects with periodontal disease are at a significantly increased risk of developing lung cancer.[49]

Periodontitis and Neurological/ Psychiatric Disease

Alzheimer's Disease

Aside from the links between periodontitis and stroke, other diseases more directly related to tissues of the brain and neurological system also have clear connections to periodontitis. Periodontal pathogens, along with other pathogens, have been linked to Alzheimer's disease, as well as to an increased cognitive decline in this disease.[50-54] Other studies have shown that elevated antibody levels to periodontal pathogens were present in Alzheimer's patients years before the presence of cognitive impairment. This finding suggests a contributory role of periodontitis with both the onset and the evolution of Alzheimer's disease.[55,56] Compromised oral hygiene, particularly with regard to peridontitis, appeared to be more prominent in nursing home patients suffering from dementia.[57] Poor oral health in general, of which periodontitis is a significant part, is also associated with various mental illnesses.[58-60] Higher cognitive function has also been associated with a lesser chance of periodontal disease.[61]

> *Periodontal pathogens, along with other pathogens, have been linked to Alzheimer's disease, as well as to an increased cognitive decline in this disease.*

Parkinson's Disease

Parkinson's disease is another neurological disease that appears to have a relationship to periodontitis.[62-65] It would appear, however, that periodontitis is just one of a number of infections that can promote Parkinson's disease, as one study found that the composite serologic measure of exposure to six common pathogens correlated as well with the development of this disease. Antibody responses to a greater number of these pathogens, consistent with a greater infectious burden, indicated a greater association with the disease.[66]

Other Neurological and Psychiatric Associations

Periodontal disease has been positively correlated with the severity of seizures in patients who don't respond to attempted treatment.[67] Depression is another neuropsychiatric disease that has a relationship to periodontitis. It has been shown that periodontal disease is an independent risk factor for the development of depression.[68] One opinion paper makes the case that depression and periodontitis both affect the development of each other. Depression appears to be a cause for periodontal disease, and periodontal disease appears to be a cause for depression.[69]

Disease associations with periodontitis that have not been as well established or extensively researched as those above but have been suggested to be significant by some researchers include multiple sclerosis and Huntington's disease.[70,71]

Periodontitis and All-Cause Mortality

Aside from being a risk factor for coronary heart disease, cancer, and neurological diseases, periodontal disease is also associated with increased all-cause mortality.[72-76]

Periodontitis is known to increase oxidative stress throughout the body, allowing it to play its role in worsening any given disease and leading to earlier death. It is likely that this reality is the reason periodontitis is linked to an increase of all-cause mortality.

In addition, research shows a correlation between the depth of periodontal pockets (indicating more detachment between the tooth and the gums) and a greater incidence of a wide variety of medical conditions.[77] Furthermore, periodontal disease has been shown to involve combinations

Aside from being a risk factor for coronary heart disease, cancer, and neurological diseases, periodontal disease is also associated with increased all-cause mortality.

of over 700 different bacterial species, along with viruses, protozoa, and fungi, all helping to set the stage for a wide array of clinical conditions.[78] When the bacterial burden of the periodontal disease is higher, the risk of angina and heart attack is higher as well.[79]

When any factor increases all-cause mortality, it means that it is inflicting a pathological effect equally on all of the cells in the body. Unless all the cells of the body are equally impacted, the mortality associated with some diseases will be impacted more than others. In the case of periodontitis, this is a generalized increase in oxidative stress secondary to the circulating factors of chronic inflammation, equally impacting all tissues and all cells. All chronic diseases share the common denominator of increased intracellular, and often extracellular, oxidative stress, which is always the manifestation of chronic inflammation.[80] Anything that can nonspecifically stimulate this generalized condition of increased oxidative stress increases all-cause mortality, and anything that can uniformly decrease it will decrease all-cause mortality. A vitamin C-rich diet and/or supplementation with vitamin C to the point of chronically sustaining higher blood levels of this vital antioxidant reliably decreases all-cause mortality. This measurable decrease is consistent with the model that posits that increased oxidative stress is actually the cause for all disease.[81-85]

Periodontitis and Other Diseases and Medical Conditions

Metabolic Syndrome

Consistent with the cause-and-effect relationship between periodontal disease and coronary heart disease, a very strong connection is also seen between periodontal disease and metabolic syndrome.[86-88] Metabolic syndrome encompasses the laboratory findings of elevated glucose, triglycerides, and total cholesterol, along with low levels of high-density lipoprotein cholesterol. This is often accompanied by hypertension, all of which makes metabolic syndrome a strong risk factor for coronary heart disease. As an elevated glucose is often part of metabolic syndrome, it also follows that periodontal disease is independently linked to diabetes. As further confirmation of this link, studies indicate that effective periodontal treatment can improve blood sugar control.[89-91]

There is a strong likelihood that the relationship of periodontitis and metabolic syndrome is one of cause-and-effect, as one study found that patients with metabolic syndrome had more severe and extensive periodontal disease compared to subjects without metabolic syndrome.[92] Furthermore, another study showed that the effective treatment of periodontal disease was able to improve total cholesterol and low-density lipoprotein cholesterol levels—two of the important laboratory parameters that are abnormal in metabolic syndrome.[93,94]

...another study showed that the effective treatment of periodontal disease was able to improve total cholesterol and low-density lipoprotein cholesterol levels...

Hypertension (High Blood Pressure)

The earliest stages of hypertension, as reflected by examining worsening parameters of arterial stiffness, compliance, and vascular endothelial function, were worse in patients with severe periodontal disease.[95] Chronic periodontitis is also associated with increased central and systemic blood pressure, along with the resulting secondary increase in left ventricular mass.[96] Additionally, periodontitis was very prevalent in a study with self-reported hypertension.[97] Another study showed that periodontitis in its more advanced forms ("destructive") was associated with even higher systolic blood pressures.[98] Periodontal disease has also been linked to an increased mortality risk in hypertensive patients.[99]

Cerebrovascular Disease

A study cited above[19] demonstrated the presence of oral pathogen DNA, including from typical periodontal species, in the tissue of ruptured intracranial aneurysms. It should come as no surprise, then, that it has been shown that periodontal disease is associated with the development of early atherosclerotic carotid lesions, a condition that would be expected to often predate the development of a stroke.[100] Later, it was shown by PCR testing that periodontal bacteria DNA is present in carotid atheromatous plaque specimens.[101] Multiple studies have documented clear and strong associations between periodontal disease and ischemic stroke.[102,103] Chronic periodontitis was also found to be independently associated with lacunar strokes after adjusting for well-known vascular risk factors.[104] Other investigators have found that a history of periodontitis is significantly associated with the incidence of cerebrovascular disease defined as stroke or transient ischemic attack.[105]

Finally, another study showed that the degree of periodontitis was important in determining the degree of the cerebrovascular disease. Researchers reported greater neurological deficit in stroke patients with advanced periodontitis at the time of admission to the hospital.[106]

Vascular Disease

As the DNA of periodontal pathogens has been found in brain aneurysms, carotid artery plaque, and coronary artery plaque, it should be expected that evidence of this oral infection would be found elsewhere in the vascular system. And that is exactly the case. Periodontal bacteria have been linked to Buerger's disease, a peripheral vascular occlusive disease seen mostly in young smokers, as well as to varicose veins, the walls of abdominal aortic aneurysms, and peripheral arterial disease in general.[107-110] A case report even demonstrated that severe chronic periodontitis was the likely cause of a septic pulmonary embolism.[111]

Pulmonary Disease

Several studies have demonstrated a significant relationship between periodontitis and pneumonia. One research group showed that patients with periodontitis were three times as likely to acquire a hospital-associated (nosocomial) pneumonia as patients without periodontitis.[112] Other researchers not only found a strong similarity between the microbiology of periodontal infection and lung infection, they also found that recurrent lung infection was effectively prevented by effectively treating the periodontal infection.[113]

...it appears that effective periodontal therapy in patients with COPD and chronic periodontitis can improve lung function and decrease the frequency of COPD exacerbations.

Chronic obstructive pulmonary disease (COPD) also appears to have a relationship with periodontitis.[114,115] Patients with more severe degrees of COPD were found to be more likely to have more severe periodontal disease.[116-118] Also, it appears that effective periodontal therapy in patients with COPD and chronic periodontitis can improve lung function and decrease the frequency of COPD exacerbations.[119,120] The relationship between COPD and periodontal disease has also been examined from a reverse perspective, finding that COPD was an independent risk factor for poor periodontal health.[121]

Chronic periodontitis also has been found to have a higher frequency in individuals with severe asthma. In one study, individuals with periodontal infection demonstrated a 5-fold greater likelihood of having bronchial inflammation than those without such infection.[122] Such inflammation would be expected to increase the incidence and degree of bronchospasm that would be seen in severe asthmatics.

Arthritis

Rheumatoid arthritis (RA), has been very strongly linked to periodontitis.[123-125] Both periodontitis and RA are chronic inflammatory diseases, with tissue damage occurring in the mouth and in the joints by similar mechanisms.[126-129] DNA from common periodontal pathogens as well as antibodies to these pathogens has been found in both the blood and in the synovial fluids of RA patients, and the pathogens appear to directly impact the autoreactivity of RA.[130-132] Studies have also shown that effective periodontal treatment consistently decreased the severity of both the RA and the periodontitis, both clinically and on abnormal laboratory parameters.[133-135] Periodontitis as a risk factor also appears to predate many cases of RA, appearing to play a prominent role in the development of this disease.[136]

Periodontitis as a risk factor also appears to predate many cases of RA, appearing to play a prominent role in the development of this disease.

Recent studies also indicate associations between periodontitis and other forms of arthritis, including juvenile idiopathic arthritis, osteoarthritis, spondyloarthritis, and psoriatic arthritis, as well as psoriasis itself.[137-140] Periodontal pathogens were detected in aspirates from the knees of osteoarthritis patients who had no history of orthopedic implants.[141]

Miscellaneous Medical Conditions

Associations have been established between periodontitis and the following medical conditions:

- ✓ Osteoporosis[142-148]
- ✓ Diabetes[149-151]
- ✓ Osteonecrosis of the jawbone[152-154]
- ✓ Prostatitis and prostate-specific antigen (PSA) levels[155]
- ✓ HIV infection[156-158]
- ✓ Systemic lupus erythematosus[159-164]
- ✓ Abnormal calcification in blood vessels and heart[165-169]
- ✓ Inflammatory bowel disease [Crohn's disease, chronic ulcerative colitis][170-173]
- ✓ Preeclampsia, maternal hypertension, maternal anemia, low birth weight, preterm birth[174-181]
- ✓ Anemia of chronic disease[182-186]
- ✓ Chronic kidney disease[187,188]
- ✓ Sudden hearing loss[189]

✓ Erectile dysfunction[190,191]
✓ Body-wide increased oxidative stress
  biomarkers [Increased parameters of
  systemic inflammation][192-200]

Conclusion

Oral infections, usually chronic periodontal disease and root canal-treated teeth, are clearly and strongly linked to a very large and diverse number of medical conditions and chronic degenerative diseases. Furthermore, evidence now clearly establishes that the oral pathogens typically seen in chronic periodontal disease and root canal-treated teeth are nearly always the ___cause___ of most heart attacks. And very good, although less compelling, evidence published to date indicates that these same pathogens with their associated toxins chronically increase oxidative stress in the breast tissues and appear to be the main cause for most cases of breast cancer.

Periodontal disease specifically is strongly correlated with, and probably causes, most significant medical conditions in most people. The dental and radiological entity known as chronic apical periodontitis (CAP) is usually asymptomatic and painless, yet it is a very advanced form of the less complicated simple and moderate forms of periodontitis already shown to be strongly correlated with so many medical conditions. The straightforward and overwhelmingly important conclusion to be taken from all of this is that the painless CAP tooth that is very prevalent in the population accounts for all the diseases associated with less advanced forms of periodontitis, yet it will usually be undetected unless specifically looked for with sophisticated X-ray imaging (3D cone beam imaging). Therefore, undiagnosed CAP teeth represent the ___**Hidden** **Epidemic**___, *and along with many poorly performed root canal-treated teeth, cause the majority of life-threatening diseases across the planet today.*

Increased Oxidative Stress: The Common Cause of All Diseases

Overview

All living systems require a continual exchange of electrons between biomolecules in order to function. This exchange is called reduction-oxidation (redox) and it occurs as one molecule takes one or more electrons from another molecule. The receipt of electron(s) by a biomolecule is called reduction and the loss of electron(s) by a biomolecule is called oxidation. A molecule cannot receive electrons unless another molecule loses them — one cannot happen without the other. In other words, redox requires one molecule to be oxidized so that another can be reduced.

Some chronic oxidation is a normal byproduct of all metabolic activity. But in healthy cells the oxidation is counterbalanced by antioxidants. Antioxidants ensure a healthy flow/supply of electrons as they reduce oxidized biomolecules by donating electrons. When antioxidant supplies become depleted, or when oxidation is occurring faster than the antioxidant system can neutralize, an abnormally high level of oxidized biomolecules results.

The state of disequilibrium caused by an excessive number of oxidized biomolecules, both inside and outside the cells, is called ***increased oxidative stress (IOS)***. The presence of IOS means that the high level of oxidized biomolecules present in a given group of cells is negatively impacting cellular function. Biomolecules include enzymes, proteins, sugars, lipids, and even nucleic acids. They can be part of the cellular structure, bound to other biomolecules, or roaming free in solution. When a biomolecule becomes oxidized, its biological function may be decreased to some degree or completely absent, depending on the biomolecule.

> *When a biomolecule becomes oxidized, its biological function may be decreased to some degree or completely absent, depending on the biomolecule.*

The presence of transition metal ions, like iron and copper, makes IOS even more pronounced since these agents are able to ramp up the production of the hydroxyl radical via the Fenton reaction.[1-3] This radical is the most reactive redox molecule known to science. It is so reactive that the moment a hydroxyl molecule is formed it will immediately oxidize any adjacent biomolecule.[4-6]

The consistent common denominator of all diseases is the presence of IOS. And the lessening or resolution of that IOS is the key to the effective treatment of all disease. IOS is literally the single parameter that determines whether a cell or tissue is diseased. When no IOS is present, no disease is present. It's that simple.

The actual diagnosis and management of any chronic disease is considerably more complex. First, it is necessary to identify the specific causes of the IOS, and then the medical practitioner must find and employ effective means to mitigate those causes. Since the causes of IOS often come from multiple sources, failure to identify one chronic source—an undiagnosed oral infection, for example—means that treatment will be only partially effective or fail altogether.

What causes IOS? The answer is simple: toxins.

The Consistent Cause of All IOS

What causes IOS? The answer is simple: toxins. Toxins are always pro-oxidant in their impact. They always, directly or indirectly, take electrons from biomolecules, either through a direct oxidation or by initiating one or more biochemical reactions that result in oxidation.

Any free radical, pro-oxidant, or other molecule that produces an increase in oxidative stress is, by virtue of its activity, a toxin. In fact, the "toxicity" of a toxin is **_nothing more_** than the degree to which it can cause biomolecules to become oxidized and to remain so.

Antioxidant = Antitoxin

Because the toxicity of all toxins is due to the depletion of electrons in the affected biomolecules, it follows that antioxidants are the ultimate antitoxins because they donate electrons (reduction), sometimes directly to the electron-seeking toxins and sometimes just restoring a full complement of electrons to previously oxidized biomolecules, restoring their normal function. When an electron-seeking toxin receives its full complement of electrons, as from an antioxidant molecule, it loses its toxicity, since it cannot any longer take electrons from another molecule. This clear-cut and very potent antitoxin effect of all antioxidants remains little appreciated by mainstream medicine, as well as by much of integrative or complementary medicine. In fact, vitamin C, the prototypical antioxidant, has been documented to be a highly effective antitoxin against all toxins, or poisons, with which it has been tested. This includes *in vitro* and *in vivo* studies in plants, animals, and humans, as well as a wide variety of clinical studies.[7,8]

Indeed, the modern poison control center need not exist at all, except to promptly administer high doses of vitamin C intravenously and orally, along with other selected antioxidant nutrients. The center could serve a role in evacuating the stomach of orally ingested toxins/poisons, along with the administration of an agent such as activated charcoal to bind and neutralize toxins still unabsorbed in the gastrointestinal tract. The administration of many antisera or species-specific antidotes, traditionally given after such events as a poisonous snakebite, often inflict their own additional toxicity and can harm as well as benefit the patient. Frederick Klenner, MD described treating a child with tetanus

> *The effects of any pro-oxidant and any toxin at the molecular level are the same: they both cause, directly or indirectly, the oxidation of various biomolecules, and they result in IOS...*

in conjunction with another physician and having to deal with the pronounced toxicity of the tetanus antitoxin doses that consistently appeared to work against the improvement seen after each intravenous vitamin C dose. Klenner also commented in this article that "massive doses of vitamin C" were "dramatically effective" in dealing with hundreds of poisonings and viral infections.[9]

The effects of any pro-oxidant and any toxin at the molecular level are the same: they both cause, directly or indirectly, the oxidation of various biomolecules, and they result in IOS in the affected cells and tissues. As noted above, an antioxidant like vitamin C is a powerful antitoxin, since it will often directly neutralize the toxin, but also because it will always help to repair oxidized biomolecules. The best antisera or species-specific antidotes will never repair the damage already done by toxin, venom, or poison. They can only help to prevent the toxin from inflicting further oxidative damage, with the hope that the patient is not too far gone for the body to overcome the damage already done and to heal itself.

Antioxidant versus Reduced Toxin

The chemical nature of a toxin prevents redonation of the electrons taken in the oxidation of biomolecules. This is a basic difference between an antioxidant and a reduced toxin, both of which have a full complement of electrons. Because of this characteristic, an antioxidant such as vitamin C promotes electron exchange and flow, while the toxin molecules generally block electron exchange and flow. This is also why an antioxidant can repair an oxidized biomolecule, while a reduced toxin cannot. Although both the antioxidant and the reduced toxin have enough electrons to give them to an electron-deficient molecule, the chemical nature of the toxin only allows it to ***take and keep*** electrons. When a toxin acquires electrons, it becomes more chemically stable and holds onto the electrons relatively tightly, unlike the antioxidant molecule, which is not markedly more chemically stable in either its reduced or oxidized form.

Cellular Electricity

As noted directly above, the chemical stability of an antioxidant such as vitamin C is similar with or without a full complement of electrons. Because of this property, vitamin C gives and takes electrons, over and over. This contributes to a real electron flow inside cells that is manifest as microcurrents, while helping to facilitate the maintenance of healthy transmembrane electrical potentials (voltages). At rest, most cell membrane potentials range from -40 to -70 millivolts. Toxic, diseased cells have lower transmembrane voltages and lesser microcurrents. The importance of these microcurrents to the health of the cell is supported by many studies that show that the application of microcurrents to injured tissue can stimulate stem cell activity and promote healing.[10,11] Multiple membrane channels regulating

> *Toxic, diseased cells have lower transmembrane voltages and lesser microcurrents.*

the flow of calcium, sodium, and potassium ions are known as "voltage-gated" membrane channels and further contribute to cellular microcurrents.[12-14] As calcium levels increase inside cells, oxidative stress is upregulated inside those cells, further impairing their ability to function normally and directly promoting all chronic diseases.[15]

Different Toxin, Different Disease

Even though the final common pathological denominator of all chronic degenerative diseases is increased oxidative stress (IOS), multiple factors affect how the IOS clinically impacts the body. Factors that figure prominently in the variability of disease expression resulting from IOS include the following:

1. **Degree of the IOS**. IOS can vary widely in actual quantity, anywhere from minimal to massive.

2. **Chronicity of the IOS**. The circumstances can be acute and "one-time" or the conditions promoting ongoing IOS can be chronic and unremitting.

3. **Location of the IOS**. This includes extracellular, intracellular (cytoplasm), intracellular organelles (endoplasmic reticula, mitochondria), cellular nuclei, and cellular groupings (organ, tissue, or compartment).

4. **Genetic predispositions** in a given patient. If an enzyme is absent, deficient, or already oxidized, this represents an area in the body where the additional oxidative stress of a new toxin can have an even greater negative clinical impact.

5. **Biochemical properties** of the pro-oxidant molecules (toxins) that are promoting the IOS. Some of the more significant variables characterizing different toxins will be examined below.

...the degree to which a tissue, organ, or a specific microenvironment in the body is optimally functional (healthy) is directly related to the ratio of how many biomolecules are reduced to how many biomolecules are oxidized...

6. **Unique combination** of the above five factors. Severe IOS resulting from the chronic exposure to a potent toxin in a particular organ might result in malignancy. On the other hand, mild intracellular and/or extracellular IOS in the muscles and joints could result in myalgias and arthralgias, but not necessarily an advanced disease.

Generally, the biomolecules of the body exist in either a reduced (electron-saturated) or an oxidized (electron-depleted) state. Rarely, a biomolecule might act as if it were chemically inert and be intrinsically resistant to oxidation. However, technically it would still be in a reduced state since it would have a full contingent of electrons.

When reduced, the biomolecules are in their state of optimal physiological function. Oxidized biomolecules exhibit decreased to absent physiological function. Therefore, the degree to which a tissue, organ, or a specific microenvironment in the body is optimally functional (healthy) is directly related to the ratio of how many biomolecules are reduced to how many biomolecules are oxidized (reduction/oxidation). A higher redox ratio will reliably reflect better physiological function and health, while lower ratios will reflect differing degrees of disease. When a toxin results in the oxidation of extremely critical biomolecules, relatively severe disease and even death can result even though the overall redox ratio in the body is relatively good.

...the biochemical nature of the pro-oxidant agent, or toxin, plays a very large role in determining the clinical relevance of the IOS that is produced and what type of disease will result.

Cyanide poisoning would be a good example of this, as this toxin rapidly inactivates critical biomolecules needed to incorporate oxygen into metabolic pathways, even though the total amount of toxin and the total number of oxidized biomolecules are relatively small compared to much less clinically potent toxins.[16]

Item #5 noted above, the biochemical nature of the pro-oxidant agent, or toxin, plays a very large role in determining the clinical relevance of the IOS that is produced and what type of disease will result. Some of the most significant properties characterizing the nature of the toxin include the following:

- ✓ **Solubility properties**. The toxin can be fat-soluble, water-soluble, or to some degree soluble in both fat and water (amphipathic).
- ✓ **Molecular size**. The toxin can be a very small molecule with easy physical access to both intracellular and extracellular areas, or it can be a very large, complex molecule that only accesses a very limited number of areas.
- ✓ **Electrical state**. Neutral or ionically charged. This characteristic not only affects where the toxin has physical access, it also impacts the degree of chemical reactivity of the toxin.

✓ **Unique molecular structure** of the toxin. The physical configuration of a toxin, especially one with a higher molecular weight and extended branches that fold in a specific spacial manner, dictates the ability of the toxin to fit in a certain manner with target biomolecules, as in a lock-and-key relationship.

✓ **Direct impact of the oxidized biomolecule(s) on biochemical functions**. One toxin might preferentially cause the oxidation of a relatively unimportant biomolecule, while another could cause the oxidation of one or more very critical biomolecules, such as those directly involved in energy production in the cell.

✓ **Tendency to produce oxidative chain reactions**. When the toxin preferentially oxidizes and inactivates critical antioxidant enzymes, the resulting increased oxidative stress can be further magnified.

✓ **Chemical reactivity of the toxin**. A chemical reaction can proceed very slowly or very rapidly, depending on the stability of the chemical configuration of the toxin. A toxin that requires a number of necessary chemical parameters to react with biomolecules in a given microenvironment will have a different clinical impact than one that reacts instantaneously, like the hydroxyl radical noted above.

✓ **Tendency to accumulate**. Some toxins can build up physical stores inside cells and elsewhere. Even when the oxidative damage has already been inflicted, a sizeable accumulation of a toxin can physically impair or even prevent biomolecules from having needed interactions, serving to further block normal biological function.

✓ **Physical similarity to biomolecules**. Some toxins can have enough physical similarities to particular biomolecules that they can act as inactive substitutes for those biomolecules, thereby decreasing the degree of normal function that would otherwise be present. Important receptors could be bound by certain toxins and rendered nonfunctional, as when a blank key fits a lock but will not open it.

✓ **Ease of access to excretion and elimination**. Whether a toxin is intracellular, extracellular, bound to other molecules, existing freely in solution, or sequestered in various storage sites helps determine how readily that toxin can be mobilized, chelated, and/or excreted.

Cancer cells, in particular, have the highest intracellular levels of IOS, and that IOS has been shown to play a role in the malignant transformation of those cells.

Levels of Intracellular Oxidative Stress

The basic metabolism of all cells results in metabolic byproducts that are pro-oxidant, and therefore toxic, in nature. As oxygen is processed and energy-rich molecules like ATP (adenosine triphosphate) are produced, waste products result as well. The degree of this oxidative stress can be of a physiologically normal degree, or it can be increased to various degrees. This depends on the type of cell and the level of its baseline metabolism, whether it is normal or already diseased, and on the amount of ongoing new toxin exposure. Of particular interest clinically is that all diseased cells demonstrate increased oxidative stress (IOS), especially intracellularly. Cancer cells, in particular, have the highest intracellular levels of IOS, and IOS has been shown to play a critical role in the malignant transformation of those cells.[17] At least eight levels of intracellular oxidative stress can exist over the spectrum of normal, diseased, and cancerous cells:

1. **Absent or non-detectable** oxidative stress, as might be found in fully differentiated, non-replicating, and dormant cells

2. **Minimal** oxidative stress, as in cells with physiological levels of baseline metabolic activity

3. **Minimal to moderate** oxidative stress, intermittently upregulated. This level is present most of the time in normally functioning, non-diseased cells that are utilizing the physiological degrees of oxidative stress being produced in multiple intracellular signaling functions, upregulating or downregulating various metabolic reactions.[18]

4. **Moderate** oxidative stress, chronically upregulated. While this level of oxidative stress can exist in a normal cell, this is usually the case only when this moderate degree is present transiently, as when a temporary burst of increased metabolic activity or energy is needed. When it is present most or all of the time, the cell can be characterized as being chronically diseased, with the stage being set for the cell to undergo malignant transformation if the intracellular

oxidative stress is pushed any higher, in concert with the presence of other carcinogenic cofactors.

5. **Moderate to elevated** oxidative stress. When chronic, this is a level of oxidative stress inside the cells that is characteristic of established and replicating cancer cells.[19] It is never found on a chronic basis inside normal cells, and it may also be present at times in chronically diseased but non-malignant cells that can easily be pushed into malignant transformation.[20,21] When oxidative stress is high enough and prolonged enough, DNA damage can occur which then further promotes malignant transformation.[22]

6. **Elevated** oxidative stress. This level of intracellular oxidative stress in seen in the most metabolically active of cancer cells, such as actively metastasizing cells, as well as in anaplastic, largely undifferentiated cancer cells.[23] Since very high levels of intracellular oxidative stress are needed for a cell to die, this level of intracellular oxidative stress can also be briefly seen in an otherwise normal cell that is rapidly upregulating its oxidative stress in order to achieve programmed cell death, or apoptosis.

7. **Greatly elevated** oxidative stress. This is the level seen in cancer cells proceeding to apoptosis or even frank necrosis, as when the Fenton reaction in the cytoplasm has been upregulated by pro-oxidant agents, such as chemotherapy.[24,25]

8. **Maximal** oxidative stress. This is the level of intracellular oxidative stress that is so elevated that the structural components of the cell are sufficiently oxidized to the degree that the physical integrity of the cell can no longer be maintained, and frank rupture occurs. This degree of oxidative stress can also exist in a previously normal or just chronically diseased cell acutely exposed to a very large toxin dose capable of inflicting enough intracellular oxidative stress to proceed directly to widespread cellular necrosis and rupture.

Conclusion

Increased oxidative stress, especially intracellularly, is the final common denominator in all chronic degenerative diseases, including heart disease and cancer. All pro-oxidant molecules are toxins, and all toxins inflict their damage by increasing the number of oxidized biomolecules. Pathogens are a major source of increased oxidative stress. All chronic infections strongly promote oxidative stress via associated endotoxins, exotoxins, and a wide variety of pro-oxidant metabolic byproducts are produced as tissue is damaged and also as pathogens eventually die and break down.

Although the cause of all disease is ultimately increased oxidative stress, the wide variety of diseases can be explained by various characteristics of the increased oxidative stress, as well as by the many different chemical characteristics of the offending pro-oxidants involved in producing the increased oxidative stress present in a given clinical syndrome or disease. Also, the degree to which intracellular oxidative stress is increased plays a major role in malignant transformation as well as in how invasive a given cancer might be.

Sources of Increased Oxidative Stress

Overview

Since increased oxidative stress (IOS) is the reason for all chronic diseases, it follows that anything that promotes increased pro-oxidant/toxin exposure is an important promoter of chronic diseases as well. In most cases, if all toxins and toxin facilitators were to be eliminated, the body would be truly freed to live a normal lifespan. Physiologically speaking, the normal lifespan would be determined by the gradual cumulative impact of the oxidative stress associated with normal cellular metabolic function. Ultimately, this would lead to tissue/organ breakdown, disease, and death.[1,2]

Exogenous Toxin Sources

Environmental Exposure

Much oxidative stress generated in the body comes from an exposure to toxins originating outside of the body. Such exposures can be acute in nature and anywhere from minimal to massive in degree. Toxin exposures can also be chronic in nature, often originating from their recurrent presence in air, food, and water or from other sources encountered on a regular basis.

Many do not realize that a large number of their other prescription drugs also have some toxicity and will inflict their own oxidative damage to the body.

Generally, most patients living under given circumstances have similar exogenous toxin exposure profiles. However, it is very important to discover whether a given patient is routinely subjected to a uniquely high toxin exposure of a certain type. For example, a farmer might have a very large pesticide exposure, and a complete success in treating that individual's health problems will likely fall far short of the mark if this ongoing toxin exposure is not accurately identified and addressed.

Inadvertent Toxin Ingestion

This category refers to the ingestion of toxins of which the individual is generally unaware. Toxicity of this type can be due to the inherent toxic nature of the substance or due to the fact that it is being overdosed. Many prescription drugs, especially chemotherapy agents, are very toxic and can profoundly increase oxidative stress in all areas of the body. Although cancerous tissues are the intended target of these agents, healthy tissues are also exposed and subjected to the increased oxidative stress they promote. While most people know that chemotherapy is toxic, many do not realize that a large number of their other prescription drugs also have some toxicity and will inflict their own oxidative damage to the body.

FAT-SOLUBLE VITAMINS

Supplementation with vitamins, minerals, and other antioxidant nutrients are generally free of significant toxicity at most dosages. However, there are a few noteworthy exceptions. Of the four fat-soluble vitamins (A, D, E, and K), three (A, D, and E) can be reliably pushed to toxic levels, as they become increasingly concentrated in the liver and fatty tissues of the body. Excess vitamin A can produce toxic effects in the liver and in the central nervous system.[3-5]

Of the four fat-soluble vitamins, three can be reliably pushed to toxic levels, as they become increasingly concentrated in the liver and fatty tissues of the body.

Vitamin D supplementation needs to be regulated in coordination with periodic testing of blood levels. Neither too little vitamin D nor too much vitamin D is desirable, as low levels are associated with increased all-cause mortality and very high levels are also very toxic.[6-8] Generally, a blood level of 50 to 80 ng/cc is the target range for optimal vitamin D benefits. Higher levels may end up proving to be beneficial, but lower levels are never desirable.

> *Even though fat-soluble, a toxic level for vitamin K supplementation has yet to be defined.*

Most doses of vitamin E are well-tolerated, but relatively rare reports have shown that it can be pushed to toxic levels in humans and animals.[9,10] However, even though fat-soluble, a toxic level for vitamin K supplementation has yet to be defined. In fact, an animal study that pushed the dosing of vitamin K to astronomical levels showed no evidence of toxicity.[11]

WATER-SOLUBLE VITAMINS

As a group, the water-soluble vitamins are almost completely nontoxic. Unlike the fat-soluble vitamins, which can accumulate in fatty tissues and in the liver, none of the water-soluble group is significantly stored in the body. Instead, they are continuously excreted in the urine, and they must be ingested on a regular basis to avoid deficiencies from developing. Largely because of this, it is difficult to supplement any of them to the point of reaching a clinically toxic level in the body.

The water-soluble vitamins include the B vitamins and vitamin C. The B vitamins are traditionally known as the vitamin B-complex group. These vitamins are thiamine (vitamin B1), riboflavin (vitamin B2), niacin (vitamin B3), pyridoxine (vitamin B6), cobalamin (vitamin B12), folate, biotin, and pantothenic acid. In the B vitamin group, even though some liver toxicity has been reported with the excess dosing of niacin, other reports demonstrate that niacin can not only protect the liver but also help resolve the condition of fatty liver.[12-15] Rare neurotoxic damage has also been reported with pyridoxine, although pyridoxine has also been documented to have a protective effect against neuropathy.[16-18] The other B vitamins have no clearly established levels of toxic intake.

Vitamin C, arguably the most important of the water-soluble vitamins, also has no established toxic level.

Vitamin C, arguably the most important of the water-soluble vitamins, also has no established toxic level. Practically the only circumstance under which vitamin C can even rarely result in undesirable side effects is when there is pre-existing renal failure or advanced renal insufficiency. This lack of toxicity is the case even when extraordinarily high doses are administered to gravely ill patients by intravenous infusion.[19] However, when allowed to accumulate in an unchecked fashion by the presence of kidney failure and decreased to absent urine output, just about all water-soluble medicines or supplements can present a potential problem.

To further put the nontoxic nature of vitamin C and the water-soluble vitamins in perspective, consider the established toxicity of water. While most people would not think of water as having the capability of being toxic, it is well-established that the deliberate ingestion of large volumes of water reliably results in a syndrome of water intoxication and even death. This can occur in both animals and humans.[20-23] In a person with normal renal function, vitamin C has **no** established level of toxicity and has never been documented to cause death. With this information, then, one can make the case that water is certainly toxic, and vastly more toxic than vitamin C. Even when potentially toxic vitamins are deliberately taken to excess, they are much more likely to result in adverse symptoms that are tolerable and readily reversible long before reaching a point of irreversible organ damage or death.

The notion that "a little is good, so more is better" does not apply to the supplementation of minerals— there is a need to exert caution to avoid toxicity.

MINERALS

Minerals can be much more easily overdosed than any of the vitamins or other antioxidant nutrients. The notion that "a little is good, so more is better" does not apply to the supplementation of minerals—there is a need to exert caution to avoid toxicity.

However, there is one noteworthy exception: magnesium. Nearly all adults have suboptimal to significantly deficient body levels of magnesium, and the oral forms of magnesium supplementation typically fall short of the goal of normalizing these levels. Large doses of magnesium given intravenously can have toxic effects,

Oral dosing with magnesium should always be pushed to the maximum tolerable amounts, as higher magnesium levels are associated with a substantial decrease in all-cause mortality.

but oral dosing of magnesium virtually always protects the patient from magnesium toxicity, mainly because excessive oral doses reliably induce loose stools and frank diarrhea. Nevertheless, oral dosing with magnesium should always be pushed to the maximum tolerable amounts, as higher magnesium levels are associated with a substantial decrease in all-cause mortality.[24]

Without going into a mineral-by-mineral analysis, most of the other minerals can be taken to excess and result in various forms of toxic side effects. However, mineral deficiencies are quite common, and the fact that they can be over-supplemented should not deter an individual from taking at least the recommended doses on a regular basis. Testing for mineral levels in the body is always a good idea in the evaluation and management of any patient, allowing a more educated and targeted regimen of mineral supplementation in order to correct mineral deficiencies without chronic overdosing. Many diseases consume higher amount of minerals than can be covered with the routine recommended dosing, and such diseases will never be optimally managed until deficiencies are judiciously addressed.

*Although it remains one of the most supplemented substances around the world, calcium supplementation is simply **never** good for you.*

Toxic Nutrients

While all of the vitamins and minerals mentioned above are appropriate to be supplemented to some degree, three common supplements should never be taken. Calcium, iron, and copper, although absolutely essential to life and good health, all very easily transition from a beneficial intake to a toxic intake, as the margin of safety is exceedingly narrow.

NEVER SUPPLEMENT WITH CALCIUM

Although it remains one of the most supplemented substances around the world, calcium supplementation is simply ***never*** good for you. The scare of osteoporosis and its grave complications continues to keep calcium near the top of the list of commonly ingested supplements. This dangerous supplementation proceeds from a gross misunderstanding of the pathophysiology of osteoporosis by patients and their physicians. Calcium supplementation and/or increased dietary calcium intake do not decrease the incidence of osteoporotic fractures, which is the supposed goal for most individuals taking calcium supplements. However, vitamin D supplementation, the common "partner" of calcium supplementation, does decrease the risk of fracture.[25,26] When a "calcium supplementation" study touts a decrease in fracture incidence, vitamin D is invariably a "co-supplement" being taken along with the calcium.

> *This dangerous supplementation proceeds from a gross misunderstanding of the pathophysiology of osteoporosis by patients and their physicians.*

In reality, increased calcium intake reliably promotes elevated intracellular calcium levels, resulting in increased intracellular oxidative stress. And as discussed earlier, increased intracellular oxidative stress causes and promotes all of the different chronic degenerative diseases. Higher coronary artery calcium scores, which directly reflect the accumulation of calcium throughout the body from all sources of intake, are associated with increased all-cause mortality, not just increased cardiac mortality.[27]

Women with the most calcium supplementation and the highest dairy intake had substantially increased all-cause mortality...

This conclusion received solid support in a large prospective study demonstrating that women with the most calcium supplementation and the highest dairy intake had substantially increased all-cause mortality as well.[28] Conversely, it has been shown that the administration of a long-acting prescription calcium channel blocker or a nutrient mineral calcium channel blocker such as magnesium decreases all-cause mortality as intracellular calcium levels are lowered.[29-31] Not surprisingly, then, there is also a large body of evidence that indicates increased calcium intake is a significant cancer-causing factor for a large number of people.[32]

NEVER SUPPLEMENT IRON APART FROM IRON DEFICIENCY ANEMIA

Unlike calcium and magnesium, which are considered macrominerals due to the relatively larger amounts of them in the body, iron is a trace mineral (micromineral) and has a relatively small physical presence in the body. Iron is also known as a transition metal, having two ionic forms, ferrous (2+) and ferric (3+), that play a very large role in the body in relaying electrons from one biomolecule to another. This ability to readily transfer electrons makes iron a major player in ramping up the oxidizing Fenton reaction inside the cells of the body. The Fenton reaction occurs when an electron is donated to peroxide inside the cell forming the hydroxyl radical—the most vigorously oxidizing substance known to man. Much of the time this electron is supplied by ferrous ion, converting to ferric ion in the process. The more ferrous ion present, the more the activity of the Fenton reaction is stimulated, and the more the oxidative stress inside the cell is increased.[33]

Nearly all cancer cells have increased to greatly increased amounts of accumulated iron.

All of this means that very small increases in iron inside the cell can massively upregulate intracellular oxidative stress, setting the stage for virtually all chronic diseases, including cancer.[34-37] Nearly all cancer cells have increased to greatly increased amounts of accumulated iron. In fact, removing iron from cancer cells with iron chelators can often decrease or stop their proliferation and even induce cell death.[38] Increased iron in the body has also been established as a significant risk factor for having a heart attack.[39]

Supplementation with iron when the blood count is normal will only push you into progressively higher levels of oxidative stress throughout the body...

Toxic levels of iron in the body can be easily avoided by monitoring the complete blood count and the ferritin level. Although iron also plays a vital role as an essential component of hundreds of enzymes and proteins, the vast majority of iron present in the body is directly involved in the synthesis and maintenance of hemoglobin. There is not a great deal of iron turnover in the body, so as long as there is enough of it in the body to support a normal hemoglobin level there is sufficient iron to support its many other functions. Therefore, when you have a normal complete blood count, there is no need to supplement iron, period.

Supplementation with iron when the blood count is normal will only push you into progressively higher levels of oxidative stress throughout the body, directly promoting cancer, heart disease, and all of the other chronic degenerative diseases. And if the blood count is normal and the ferritin level is greater than 100 ng/cc, specific efforts should be made to bring that level down, preferably below 50 ng/cc, via blood donation, far infrared sauna sweating, and/or supplementation with a nutrient iron chelator like inositol hexaphosphate (IP6). Prescription iron chelators are also available, but it is not usually necessary to utilize these agents to bring the iron status under control. Furthermore, as long as the blood count remains normal, there need not be any concern of driving the ferritin too low. Endurance athletes can routinely drop their ferritin levels to as low as 12 ng/cc without the appearance of an iron deficiency anemia, as sweating is a reliable way to eliminate iron from the body.[40]

In the case of ferritin, then, any measurement between 30 and 400 ng/cc is actually abnormal...

One of the largest blood testing laboratories in the United States assigns a reference range for ferritin between 30 and 400 ng/cc. Not only is 400 ng/cc already a grossly elevated level of ferritin, there is clear evidence that a ferritin level of only 50 ng/cc still significantly increases oxidative stress and impairs endothelial function in the arteries of the body relative to a level between 15 and 20 ng/cc.[41] In the case of ferritin, then, any measurement between 30 and 400 ng/cc is actually abnormal, and the entire reference range exceeds the truly normal levels.

It is essential not to confuse a laboratory reference range with a laboratory normal range. What the laboratory lists as a reference range is just assumed by many to be what is also a normal range. Sometimes this is true, but many times it is not. Remember that any laboratory test ultimately derives its reference range by making sure that a substantial percentage, often a significant majority, of the population falls within that reference range. However, when most of the population shares the same chronic toxin exposures, that reference range can be largely (or completely) abnormal, as is the case with ferritin.

Virtually all processed foods have iron added to them, and consequently millions of Americans unwittingly consume excess iron on a regular basis.

With all of this reasoning in mind, it would appear that maintaining a ferritin below 30 ng/cc, the suggested lower limit of the laboratory reference range, would be the desirable goal to minimize or even prevent any excess iron-induced oxidative stress throughout the body. Cholesterol levels and C-reactive protein (CRP) levels are two other prominent examples of laboratory tests that have reference ranges with only minimal overlap into normal ranges.

Virtually all processed foods have iron added to them, and consequently millions of Americans unwittingly consume excess iron on a regular basis. As iron is not readily excreted, it then accumulates, starting with the "iron-enriched" food of infancy. This continues throughout life with all other foods labeled "enriched," which always includes unneeded iron. It is impossible for anyone to supplement correctly or even eat correctly until there is a complete understanding of what is and what is not toxic.

Quite literally, the only thing that copper supplementation accomplishes is to increase oxidative stress throughout the body.

NEVER SUPPLEMENT WITH COPPER

Copper is similar to iron as it is also a trace mineral essential to normal physiological function, yet very easily pushed to toxic levels in the body. Like iron, copper is a transition metal that plays a significant role in the relay of electrons inside the cell. Copper also upregulates the Fenton reaction inside the cell, readily resulting in excess levels of oxidative stress in the same way that iron does.

But these two minerals differ in an important nutritional aspect. While some individuals can legitimately be iron-deficient when anemia is present and require a limited course of iron supplementation, it is virtually impossible for someone to be deficient in copper. In fact, a clear clinical syndrome of copper deficiency remains to be defined.

Quite literally, the only thing that copper supplementation accomplishes is to increase oxidative stress throughout the body. Consistent with this assertion are multiple animal and human studies that have shown that copper levels inside cancer cells as well as in the circulating blood of individuals with cancer are elevated. These studies also show that both copper and iron administration promote the development of cancer.

In a nutshell, calcium and copper should never be supplemented. And iron should never be supplemented unless there is a laboratory-documented iron deficiency anemia present.

Studies also demonstrate that the highest levels of copper correlate with the most aggressive and metastatic of tumors. It has also been demonstrated that the effective removal of copper with chelation significantly suppresses tumor growth.[42-50] Similar to iron, an elevated copper level has also been established as a risk factor for having a heart attack.[51] Both copper and iron have been documented to accumulate in the atherosclerotic plaques that lead to heart attacks.[52]

Just as increased calcium intake has been documented to increase all-cause mortality, the same has been seen with iron and copper. Increased ferritin levels are associated with increased all-cause mortality.[53] And increased copper levels in the body, as measured by looking at the copper/zinc ratio in the blood, are also associated with increased all-cause mortality.[54] Viewing all of the evidence collectively, then, it is clear that to at least some degree, supplemental calcium, iron, and copper can all legitimately be considered carcinogens, as well as nonspecific promoters of chronic degenerative diseases.

In a nutshell, calcium and copper should never be supplemented. And iron should never be supplemented unless there is a laboratory-documented iron deficiency anemia present. Upon correction of the anemia, iron should then be discontinued. Admittedly, many people who take a multivitamin/multimineral supplement and report that they feel better because of it. However, when you take a supplement with many different components and seem to benefit from it, this does not mean that everything in that supplement is beneficial. Many such supplements also contain calcium, iron, and copper. If all but a few ingredients in a supplement provide a nutritional benefit, you may well feel an overall positive improvement. Nevertheless, great caution should be exercised. One or two toxic ingredients in a generally beneficial supplement can still produce a needless negative health impact, even if the sense of well-being is improved.

Endogenous Toxin Sources

Pathogens

In terms of overall public health impact, pathogens are far and away the greatest source of disease-causing toxins. At times and at certain sites the pathogens can be present in low titer and be more of a colonization or even contamination than an infection. At other times there can be a sudden and severe onset of frank infection, with an overwhelming proliferation of pathogens, as with an acute infection such as influenza. Most frequently, pathogens are in an intermediate stage of proliferation. They often sustain a chronic infection without exhibiting a discernible impact on the body, even though the negative clinical impact can be enormous.

Pathogen-related toxins often present a more pervasive threat and therefore require diligence in diagnosis and treatment.

Although a toxin from any source, as in air, food, or water can cause disease in a given person that could eventually lead to death, pathogen-related toxins often present a more pervasive threat and therefore require diligence in diagnosis and treatment. They are extremely common, extremely potent, and largely undiagnosed and unsuspected. Furthermore, they are only rarely vigorously and definitively addressed with the urgency they warrant when they are known to be present by the treating physician or dentist.

Most of the significant pathogen-related toxins come from sources in the oral cavity...

Most of the significant pathogen-related toxins come from sources in the oral cavity,[55,56] which include the following:

✓ Acutely infected and painful teeth, with pulpal involvement.

✓ Chronically infected, typically asymptomatic teeth

✓ Teeth with X-ray evidence of chronic apical periodontitis (CAP)

✓ Root canal-treated teeth, with and without X-ray evidence of CAP

✓ Mild to advanced chronic periodontal (gum) inflammation and infection

✓ Cavitational osteonecrosis, found at many old extraction sites, as well as around the root tips of CAP teeth and root canal-treated teeth, and capable

of spreading throughout much of the
jawbone and then to the body
- ✓ Chronically inflamed and infected
  implants
- ✓ Chronically infected and abscessed
  tonsils, primarily due to the chronic
  venous and lymphatic drainage of the
  oral infections noted above[57]
- ✓ Chronically infected sinuses (often
  adjacent to a chronically infected tooth
  in the upper jawbone, or maxilla)
- ✓ Chronically infected lymph nodes
  and soft tissues of the head, neck, and
  mediastinum (usually due to lymphatic/
  venous drainage of oral infections)

The term "focal infection" has been attributed
to any definable area of the body, usually quite
small, that has a concentration of pathogens, but
without evidence of a systemic, or body-wide, infectious disease. The list above represents the most
common sites of focal infection in the population,
statistically speaking.

Other sources, or foci, of infection-related toxicity outside of the oral cavity are relatively few and of statistically far less importance.
Furthermore, they often originate because of an
earlier seeding from an oral pathogen focus, and
they will frequently resolve after the elimination
of the oral focus.[58] However, when all oral infec-

tions have been successfully eradicated and chronic disease symptoms persist, a more thorough search for persistent focal infections outside of the mouth must be undertaken.

Focal infection sites outside of the oral cavity that have been documented in the past to cause or contribute to any of a variety of diseases include the following:[59]

- ✓ Bronchial tree, as chronic bronchitis with bronchiectasis[60]
- ✓ Intestinal tract, including ulcerative processes and infected hemorrhoids;[61] also diverticulitis
- ✓ Appendix, chronically infected[62]
- ✓ Mesenteric lymph glands
- ✓ Gallbladder
- ✓ Liver
- ✓ Fallopian tubes and/or uterus, often after miscarriage or post-delivery
- ✓ Prostate gland, urethral tract, and/or seminal vesicles
- ✓ Skin and related appendages (boils, furuncles, toenails)
- ✓ Heart (endocarditis)
- ✓ Kidney (often seeded from oral focal infection)[63]
- ✓ Joint (usually seeded from oral focal infection)
- ✓ Vein inflammation/infection[64]

✓ Bone inflammation/infection

Compromised Digestion

DIGESTION VERSUS PUTREFACTION

While the diet can be a source of significant exogenous toxins that are already present in
the food when eaten, poor or incomplete digestion can result in the production of a substantial,
ongoing (usually daily) source of additional toxins.
Depending on a number of different factors, the
processing status of food in your gastrointestinal
tract can fall somewhere between optimal digestion
and advanced putrefaction (rotting). Just as in the
mouth, there is a very wide array of microbes and
pathogens in the gut. So the opportunities are ever
present for poor digestion to help the normally low
percentage of pathogenic gut microbes to selectively
proliferate and produce large amounts of toxins,
further impeding good digestion.

Several significant negatives occur when digestion partially diverts to putrefaction. A portion
of the nutrient value of the ingested food never
gets assimilated. At the same time, some of the
ingested food putrifies, producing a wide variety
of toxins and toxic metabolic byproducts of both
the food and the pathogens that are proliferating.
In addition, the putrefaction process can greatly
slow down the transit time in the gut, which further
promotes more putrefaction. This also augments the

negative impact of pathogen population and associated toxins, as there is more time for toxins to be
absorbed and/or exert their toxic effects in the gut.
Furthermore, a constipated gut will be much more
supportive of the development of gastrointestinal
foci of infection, such as is seen in diverticulitis,
than when gut transit
time is normal.[65,66]

Generally speaking, a
completely normal bowel
transit time should turn
a meal into a bowel evac-
uation every 12 to 18
hours. Going without a
bowel movement for over
24 hours is an early form

*Just like oral focal
infections have long
been linked to coronary
artery disease, the
"focal infection" of
diverticular disease is
now linked to it as well.*

of constipation and can become a source of toxicity,
and going for days without a bowel movement can
make the gut a source of great toxicity. Similar
to laboratory reference ranges that need to put a
majority of the population into the "normal" range,
as with the example of ferritin discussed earlier,
some literature asserts that a total gut transit time
of three full days can still be normal, a profoundly
ridiculous assertion.[67]

As bowel transit times become prolonged,
bacterial overgrowth can develop in the small intestine and become much like a focal infection itself,[68]
even though the area involved is larger and not so
focal compared with the other sites of infection

mentioned above. And just like oral focal infections have long been linked to coronary artery disease, the "focal infection" of diverticular disease is now linked to it as well.[69] The role that the bacterial flora of the intestine can play in motility disorders is further highlighted by the fact that fecal transplantation with a healthier flora can actually shorten the gut transit time in constipated individuals.[70] It would appear, though, that the flora-constipation relationship goes both ways. Constipation can result in an abnormal flora, and an abnormal flora can promote constipation.

The typical manner of eating by most adults throughout the world shares features that reliably impede optimal digestion, slow gut transit time, and increase putrefaction. Some of the most important of these factors include the following:

✓ Insufficient chewing
✓ Too much water or other liquids during the meal (diluting digestive enzyme concentrations)
✓ Insufficient production of digestive enzymes (supplemental enzymes usually indicated)
✓ Poor food combinations (major contributors to a sluggish gut)
✓ Infrequent, large meals versus small, more frequent meals
✓ Alcohol with the meal
✓ Milk with the meal

As so many people have significant digestive problems, relatively minor problems like belching and feeling a bit bloated are just considered normal. Indeed, the many over-the-counter and prescription agents that target the symptoms of gas, heartburn, and colic are a large chunk of the healthcare industry by themselves. However, what is really normal is no gut-related symptomatology. You should eat a meal and feel completely comfortable. Most people never get to realize such an asymptomatic state after eating. The main reason for this is that eating habits are completely cultural in nature, never properly addressing what is needed to support physiologically optimal digestion.[71]

Any iron supplementation in an adult who does not have a regular source of iron loss... results in progressive iron accumulation in the body.

IRON-MEDIATED TOXICITY
TO DIGESTION

Poor digestion and digestion-related toxicity also result from the addition of iron to all enriched or fortified foods that are consumed daily throughout the world. Unfortunately, once the public health authorities in the United States implement such a policy, the rest of the developed world usually follows such a policy without question. This addition of iron to nearly all processed foods has been taking place since 1941.

As noted earlier under "Toxic Nutrients," few adults have ferritin (iron storage) levels that are not elevated. This begs the question: Why? Without undertaking specific iron-mobilizing measures or taking specific iron-chelating agents to pull iron out of the body, all but a tiny portion of one's daily intake of iron is retained in the body. As a result, any iron supplementation in an adult who does not have a regular source of iron loss, as with the bleeding associated with menstruation or a gastro-intestinal cancer, results in progressive iron accu-mulation in the body. As already discussed, this has its own significant toxicity and impact on oxidative stress throughout the body.

However, the presence of added iron to food also directly promotes chronically increased oxida-tive stress in the gastric and intestinal lining cells in the gut. Increased oxidative stress in the diges-tive tract always produces inflammation. When sufficient iron is ingested on a regular basis, this inflammation becomes chronic, and the leaky gut syndrome will reliably emerge. This increase in gut cell inflammation occurs even when the iron ingested is in a legitimate "supplemental" form, such as ferrous sulfate.

Incredibly, however, much of the iron added to "enriched" foods (usually added to the wheat flour portion of the food) is in the form of elemental iron. In other words, the iron is in the form of ***metallic filings*** that can be pulled out of many cereals and related products with water, a blender, and a strong magnet. The iron filings that are typically added to countless enriched foods are available as the waste byproduct of the grinding, filing, or milling of finished industrial iron products and would otherwise be discarded if there was not a market for putting them in food products.

Not surprisingly, iron ingested in a pure metallic form is even more toxic than a true supplemental form of iron. Even though there may occur a minimal assimilation of iron that might occur when stomach acid encounters the filings, the rest of the undissolved iron will reliably induce a foreign body reaction in whatever cells are involved in trying to process the metal. And since so many people encounter this form of iron one or more times on a daily basis, there is no opportunity for the gut to ever recover or heal, once the inflammation has been initiated. Instead, it becomes chronically inflamed. This dietary iron assault can be expected to lead directly to, or to contribute strongly to:

> *The iron filings that are typically added to countless enriched foods are available as the waste byproduct of the grinding, filing, or milling of finished industrial iron products...*

✓ Leaky gut syndrome, permitting assimilation of incompletely digested food, which will predispose to food allergies, including peanuts, along with autoimmune diseases, both with and without areas of chronic focal infection in the gut

✓ Chronic malabsorption with less nutrient intake and more putrefaction-related toxin production, as well as compromised gut-related immune cell function

✓ Gastric and duodenal ulcers, heartburn and acid reflux, gas, cramping, and diarrhea/constipation syndromes

✓ Crohn's disease and chronic ulcerative colitis

✓ Celiac sprue and gluten sensitivity/allergy

Also, all bacterial pathogens (with the exception of the Lyme pathogen) require iron to proliferate[72]— the more iron, the higher the pathogen population. This includes *Helicobacter pylori*, the pathogen currently felt to play an important role in the development of ulcers. Furthermore, consider that this iron assault on digestive tracts begins the moment the baby switches from breast to bottle. Iron "enrichment" of baby formulas is prominently marketed as a good thing. Due to the current state of misinformation in nutrition, few concerned mothers would consider buying any products that were not enriched.

It is very likely that the current proliferation of gluten allergies, sensitivities, and even outright celiac sprue (very advanced gluten sensitivity) is largely due to this continual ingestion of iron that we do not need. As mentioned, iron was first added to food in 1941. Data gathered from an Air Force study shows that celiac sprue has increased 400% since 1948 in men as they age. It may well be that gluten sensitivity is strongly promoted by, if not directly caused by, the iron-induced inflammation in the gut, allowing the resulting leaky gut to permit gluten to be assimilated largely undigested, provoking antigen-antibody and other autoimmune reactions. Gluten is likely no more toxic than a peanut when it is properly digested in the absence of a leaky, chronically-inflamed gut.

> *It is very likely that the current proliferation of gluten allergies, sensitivities, and even outright celiac sprue is largely due to this continual ingestion of iron that we do not need.*

Of note, most foods labeled "gluten-free" are also **_not_** enriched and have no added iron. Along with organic wheat products, which also usually have no added iron, a major benefit of such foods is the absence of added iron. Effectively, when you go "gluten-free," you also go "added iron-free." When iron "enrichment" in the diet can be completely eliminated, many patients with leaky gut syndromes can actually heal. When the leaky gut is not too severe and advanced in degree, this healing can take place over about a six-month period. It is certainly possible that legitimate gluten sensitivities and even peanut allergies could greatly or even completely resolve when the gut completely heals. However, it is not being recommended that individuals with such allergies should ever again deliberately ingest these substances. Certainly, many advanced syndromes associated with a leaky gut syndrome can be expected to benefit and show significant improvement as a result of avoiding the iron-enriched foods.

CHRONICALLY POOR NUTRIENT ASSIMILATION

All of this information on compromised digestion indicates that very many people, probably the vast majority, have compromised nutrient uptake and assimilation as well. The ultimate goal of an optimally organic, nutritious diet is to get the nutrient, antioxidant molecules contained in that food into the body and inside the cells to the greatest degree possible. Therefore, it is very important to get an idea as to how well nutrients are getting where they need to go in a given individual or patient.

For the younger person with no medical problems, it is difficult to convince such a person that they should do something involved to protect the good health that they have. However, for many older individuals on multiple prescription medicines and one or more chronic diseases, it is much less difficult to demonstrate to them that something further can be done. As noted above, practically all such individuals have compromised digestion and compromised abilities to get the nutrients out of food and into their cells. Many individuals make smoothies with a wide variety of nutritious components. This is a wonderful habit, to be sure, and undoubtedly improves the nutritional status of anyone who does it. However, if someone is already doing this and not feeling especially well, an additional step can be taken.

While effective detoxification can be extremely important in realizing a clinical recovery from a number of medical conditions, it is always a double-edged sword to some degree...

A device called the NutriBullet (I have no connection, financial or otherwise) appears to completely pulverize foods, nuts, and seeds in a way and to a degree that blending simply cannot. This device completely liquefies ingredients to a degree that regular blenders cannot achieve. Such Complete Food Pulverization (CFP) allows the gut to absorb and assimilate into the cells a percentage of nutrient antioxidants from food not achievable by any other approach. While it may not be a "natural" way to eat, there is nothing natural about ingesting metallic iron or having your gut poisoned by so many toxins as are encountered today. CFP allows your gut and your body to compensate for this gut damage and the many shortcomings of a modern diet. I feel strongly that anyone who does not have the perfect health they are seeking to consider adding CFP to their daily routine.

Toxin Mobilization

Another major source of endogenous toxins comes from the mobilization of toxins that had already been stored or assimilated in a tissue or organ. Detoxification always involves some degree of retoxification. Even when the toxin load can be diminished over time with effective chelators or facilitators of excretion, a percentage of the toxins that get mobilized from storage sites will nevertheless inflict new toxic oxidative stress on new tissues after being released into the extracellular fluid and blood. While effective detoxification can be extremely important in realizing a clinical recovery from a number of medical conditions, it is always a double-edged sword to some degree, and measures need to be taken to acutely protect the body from the increased oxidative stress that always results when toxins are mobilized in the course of being excreted and eliminated.

Toxin mobilization is often due to the effects of chelation. Chelating agents bind to toxins, rendering them chemically inert and allowing them to be excreted. However, when large amounts of toxins are being mobilized, a small but significant percentage of the chelate-toxin complexes can sometimes dissociate to a variable degree, allowing the freed toxin to be taken up again into the body before it can be excreted, causing the retoxification effect noted above.

There are several ways that toxins already stored in the body end up being mobilized and causing an acute increase in oxidative stress in the extracellular fluid, the blood, and sometimes in the intracellular space, or cytoplasm. Among the most important ways include the following:

✓ **Activation of endogenous chelators.** When large amounts of antioxidants are administered, such as with a multigram dose of vitamin C intravenously, previously oxidized and dormant enzyme chelators inside diseased cells can be reactivated (reduced), and a surge of effective intracellular chelation and toxin excretion can acutely take place.

✓ **Administration of exogenous chelators.** Commonly administered prescription chelators include DMPS,

DMSA, and EDTA, as well as effective nutrient chelators like inositol hexaphosphate (IP6), alpha lipoic acid, and glutathione. In the right clinical setting, such chelators can cause a surge of toxins to appear in the blood and extracellular space, causing increased oxidative stress.

✓ **Rapid killing of cancer cells**. Cancer cells are already centers of increased oxidative stress, and when they are killed and lysed, a great deal of free radicals and oxidized biomolecules are released. Furthermore, when cancer cells are lysed, a large amount of free, reactive iron is released into the extracellular space and circulation. The increase in detectable free iron in the circulation from this cancer cell death can persist for weeks, meaning antioxidant coverage and treatment for the increased oxidative stress must continue over this period of time to prevent damage to the immune system and clinical deterioration.[73-75]

✓ **Rapid killing of pathogens**. Pathogens are effectively factories of oxidative stress. Whenever they are killed quickly and in large amounts, exotoxins, endotoxins, and oxidized metabolic byproducts are released. Like cancer cells that have lysed, non-viral pathogens that have lysed release a great deal of free iron. The host cells that sustain virus growth also have increased iron levels that are released upon being effectively killed and lysed, even though the virus particles themselves do not accumulate iron.[76]

Proper hormone replacement therapy has been shown to significantly reduce the increased all-cause mortality associated with estrogen deficiency in women.

Toxin Modulators

The ability of toxins to effectively increase oxidative stress throughout the body is strongly impacted by hormonal status. Hormones, in particular estrogen, testosterone, and thyroid, are very critical factors in determining whether cellular metabolism proceeds normally and efficiently. Chronic deficiencies of estrogen in women, of testosterone in men, and of thyroid hormone in either sex are all associated with increased all-cause mortality.[77-85]

Not surprisingly, combined hormone deficiencies have the highest risk of increased all-cause mortality. Elderly men with low levels of both testosterone and estrogen had a higher risk of mortality than with a deficiency of either one alone.[86] Of note, thyroid balance in the body is especially important, since both minimal to marked degrees of both hypothyroidism and hyperthyroidism are risk factors for increased all-cause mortality.[87,88]

Even more significantly, proper hormone replacement therapy has been shown to significantly reduce the increased all-cause mortality associated with estrogen deficiency in women.[89] A large Swedish study that followed 23,346 women over a period of eight to nine years specifically found that 11 of the 12 major categories of cause of death were favorably impacted by improved estrogen status. Death due to injury, a category not generally linked to estrogen status, was the only category that was not favorably impacted.[90]

When addressing hormone replacement therapy, there are many variations in how it can be implemented clinically. Done improperly, it can certainly increase medical problems and shorten the lifespan. However, just because it can be implemented improperly and result in an increase in morbidity and mortality does not mean it should be avoided. The long-term studies clearly show a profound benefit in length and quality of life when it is administered correctly. While a topic deserving of more detailed attention, it is important here to just note that whether hormone replacement is beneficial or effectively toxic to the body relates directly to the attention paid to the following therapeutic considerations:

✓ Dose (higher, more side effects)

✓ Type (animal origin, bioidentical)

✓ Formulation (pills, gels, sprays, etc.)

✓ Other hormone administration

✓ Route of administration (oral, transdermal); transdermal always less problematic when feasible

✓ Duration of administration (possible dosage decrease over time)

✓ Timing of initial administration (more conservative protocol starting at older age)

✓ Pre-treatment hormone levels should be objectively below the range of normal, not just in the low normal range

Instituting a proper hormone replacement therapeutic protocol involves much more time and attention for the physician in charge than for most other treatments or clinical interventions.

✓ Concurrent antioxidant administration (profoundly decreasing any side effects)

✓ Serial clinical correlation (symptomatic relief)

✓ Serial laboratory testing (improving or worsening; parameters of metabolic syndrome important to be followed;

worsening of laboratory tests can predate a clinical deterioration, such as an increasing C-reactive protein)

As a good rule of thumb, without going into detail on all of the specifics of the above therapeutic considerations for administering hormone therapy, it is of paramount importance that the dose is low and that dosage increases are small and not too frequent. If possible, the hormones should be bioidentical and the target laboratory hormone levels should be low normal to mid-range normal at the most. And for individuals over the age of 70 or already with advanced states of chronic disease with minimal clinical stability, the target level should be even lower. Extra attention to these parameters should also be paid whenever treating a hormone-deficient patient with documented coronary heart disease, at any age.

Tissues with a hypothyroid status are much more easily infected, acutely and chronically, than those with a normal thyroid status.

Instituting a proper hormone replacement therapeutic protocol involves much more time and attention for the physician in charge than for most other treatments or clinical interventions. Generally, there must be an increased time investment by the clinician for the patient to consistently benefit from thyroid and sex hormone replacement therapies. Except in very rare cases, administration of a limited and carefully monitored regimen of hormone replacement therapy for an individual with markedly low hormone levels should always be undertaken.

The importance of low or diminished thyroid function deserves some additional attention, particularly with regard to its impact on focal infection and the ability of pathogens to take hold and become effectively seeded elsewhere in the body. It has already been noted that pathogens are the most important sources of significant and chronic disease-causing oxidative stress in the body. It would appear that maintaining a euthyroid (normal thyroid) status in the body provides a strong protection against the dissemination and proliferation of such pathogens, resulting in the development of distant and new focal infections. Tissues with a hypothyroid status are much more easily infected, acutely and chronically, than those with a normal thyroid status.

Tissues with a hypothyroid status are much more easily infected, acutely and chronically, than those with a normal thyroid status.

At least 90% of all patients with coronary heart disease and heart attacks have their atherosclerotic plaque growth initiated and propagated by the pathogens that disseminate from focal dental infections, particularly root canal-treated teeth and chronic gum disease. This cause-and-effect relationship was definitively proven by the identification of these pathogens in a very high concentration in the blood clots that acutely obstructed the coronary arteries and caused myocardial infarctions.[91]

Dr. Barnes also noted that at least 30 more heart attacks occurred in individuals who stopped their thyroid therapy and dropped out of the study.

Broda Barnes, MD reported on 1,569 patients that he treated with dessicated thyroid, most over a 20-year period. For a group of this size and average age, the statistics compiled in the Framingham study established that 72 individuals in such a group should have sustained heart attacks during a comparable period of time. Incredibly, only **4** men in this group had heart attacks during this period! And there were **no** heart attacks in the 844 women in this group. Deeper examination of the study further underscores the apparently profound protective effect that normal thyroid status has on preventing the pathogen colonization leading to the evolution of coronary heart disease. A majority of the men in the study group (62%) were smokers, and Dr. Barnes did not even require that smoking be stopped or that any dietary or exercise modifications be followed during the treatment period. Dr. Barnes also noted that at least 30 more heart attacks occurred in individuals who stopped their thyroid therapy and dropped out of the study.[92]

It also needs to be stressed that the large group of patients treated and followed by Dr. Barnes were not screened in any fashion as to the incidence or presence of risk factors for heart disease. As such, this group had to have had the same prevalence of root canal-treated teeth and periodontal disease, along with other important cardiac risk factors, as the rest of the population at large. As already mentioned, there were a very large number of smokers in this group as well, which virtually assures a high prevalence of significant periodontal disease.

It is important to realize that diagnosing the mild forms of hypothyroidism... require a careful clinical evaluation along with laboratory testing beyond the "standard" thyroid testing.

As noted previously, the evolution of coronary atherosclerosis that eventually leads to heart attack is frequently caused by pathogens in root canal-treated teeth and chronic gum disease that take hold in the lining of the coronary arteries and promote chronic inflammation. This suggests that these patients were **_almost completely protected_** from coronary arterial inflammation during the treatment period by maintaining a completely normal thyroid status with dessicated thyroid.

It would appear, then, that maintaining a normal thyroid status not only helps to normalize cellular metabolism throughout the body, it also lessens oxidative stress body-wide which logically plays a vital role in preventing infections from taking hold elsewhere in the body. While similar clinical observations have not been specifically made with regard to infections spreading more readily when estrogen or testosterone levels are low, it is highly likely that having normal levels of these hormones further protects against infection spread and proliferation, since both of these hormones help to lessen oxidative stress in the cells of the body.

..."low-T3 syndrome"... is consistently associated with increased oxidative stress and chronic inflammatory diseases.

It is important to realize that diagnosing the mild forms of hypothyroidism that predispose to focal infections taking hold in the coronary arteries and elsewhere in the body require a careful clinical evaluation along with laboratory testing beyond the "standard" thyroid testing. Measuring T3, T4, and TSH levels are often useful in detecting advanced degrees of hypothyroidism and just about any degree of hyperthyroidism. However, for the growing epidemic of minimal to mild hypothyroidism that is present in arguably a substantial majority of the adult population of the world, these tests routinely fail to be of much use. Often, this gives a false reassurance that thyroid function is normal.

The reason for this is that the standard thyroid testing is really only reflective of what is going on inside the thyroid gland, but not inside the cells throughout the body. The active form of thyroid hormone, T3, is converted from its precursor, T4, roughly 80 to 90% of the time in the cytoplasm of the body's cells, with the remainder of the conversion taking place in the thyroid gland.[93] Effectively, this means that if the T4 in the cytoplasm is not being efficiently converted to the active T3 form of thyroid hormone, the traditional testing could show normal thyroid gland function while the remainder of the non-thyroid cells throughout the body may actually be clinically hypothyroid. Many hypothyroid individuals have this "intracellular" form of hypothyroidism. Hypothyroidism of this type has been described in the medical literature as "low-T3 syndrome," characterized by a reduced peripheral conversion of T4 to T3 in the presence of normal thyroid hormone secretion. This syndrome is consistently associated with increased oxidative stress and chronic inflammatory diseases.[94] It can also be referred to as "tissue" hypothyroidism, versus "glandular" hypothyroidism, in which the thyroid gland is the culprit.

While the accuracy of standard thyroid laboratory testing remains questionable in the diagnosis and monitoring of much clinical hypothyroidism, some additional testing can assist the clinician a great deal in detecting, treating, and properly following such patients.

When other conditions are being treated and sources of increased oxidative stress are being eliminated or effectively managed, close monitoring of the thyroid status needs to be done.

Normally, intracellular enzymes known as deiodinases, especially the D2 form, convert the T4 supplied by the thyroid gland into the active T3 hormone inside the cell, where it can promptly exert its hormonal effects or be released into the circulation.[95] However, some of the T4 is converted into an inactive form of T3 known as reverse T3. In situations of increased oxidative stress and chronic disease, a greater amount of the inactive reverse T3 is formed rather than the active T3 hormone. Treating this condition of decreased T3 requires the administration of prescription T3 or dessicated thyroid, which contains both T3 and T4, along with doing everything else possible to relieve the state of increased oxidative stress that provoked the formation of the reverse T3 in the first place. T4 by itself, which is the most common thyroid prescription, does not reliably improve this form of hypothyroidism, since the defect is in the conversion of T4 to T3.[96]

It is essential, then, that routine blood testing includes measurements of free T3 and reverse T3. Generally, an individual has normal peripheral thyroid function and activity when the ratio of T3 to reverse T3 is at about 20 to 1. A slighter higher ratio is acceptable, but a lower ratio, such as 18 to 1 or less, generally indicates the need for some thyroid replacement therapy. Clinically, dessicated thyroid extract works well, although some patients will respond well to prescription forms of pure T3. As mentioned above, prescription T4 often does little to no good for individuals with intracellular hypothyroidism, yet it remains the most prescribed form of thyroid hormone therapy. Clinical evaluation, along with serial body temperatures as pioneered by Dr. Barnes, are also very useful in both diagnosing the patient as well as in monitoring the clinical response to therapy.

When other conditions are being treated and sources of increased oxidative stress are being eliminated or effectively managed, close monitoring of the thyroid status needs to be done. Increased systemic oxidative stress is a major player in increasing the levels of reverse T3. Therefore, when other conditions have been effectively treated, ongoing testing needs to be done to make sure that the thyroid status of the patient has not significantly improved. Under such circumstances, thyroid supplementation can be decreased and sometimes even stopped.

Conclusion

Since increased oxidative stress is at the root of all diseases, it is important to understand as precisely as possible what the main sources of increased oxidative stress are in the population today. Ultimately, toxins (pro-oxidants, free radicals) are the etiology of all excess oxidative stress, beyond the levels of oxidative stress that are produced in the normal metabolic physiological functioning of the cells throughout the body. Therefore, knowing where the primary sources of toxins are allows the development of treatment protocols that will alleviate symptoms and slow disease evolution. But sometimes these protocols can also lay the foundation for the reversal and occasional cure of chronic degenerative diseases currently regarded as completely irreversible. For the most part, mainstream medicine seeks to lessen symptoms without any meaningful attempt to identify and eliminate the reasons for the disease developing in the first place. When occult toxin-producing infections can be identified and eliminated, primary disease resolution can sometimes be seen along with just symptom resolution.

Furthermore, as the role of occult focal infections is so important in so many chronic diseases, it must be remembered that the need to normalize intracellular thyroid function is absolutely vital to preventing/minimizing the metastasis or dissemination of such infections. Addressing this epidemic of minimal hypothyroidism in so many individuals is arguably one of the most important yet typically unaddressed factors in minimizing heart disease and most chronic degenerative diseases, including cancer. Similarly, objectively low sex hormone levels must be identified and effectively treated.

Tooth and Gum Infections

Overview

The oral cavity provides the perfect environment for the growth of microorganisms, and well over 500 different species of bacterial, viral, and fungal microbes have been documented to grow there. Even when there is no sign of a clinical problem or an overt manifestation of infection, oral pathogens are always being harbored in the mouth. So it should come as no surprise that the mouth is a very common site to find localized (focal) infections. Whenever a significant immune challenge is encountered, these sites of minimal pathogen colonization can quickly proliferate into thriving colonies. All that is required is something as simple as an acute exposure to a high titer of pathogens (such as airplane air or someone sneezing in your face) and/or a compromise in your immune defenses for various reasons (such as significant acute or chronic toxin exposures).

The most common, and the most clinically consequential, oral cavity sites of infection are the teeth, the gums, the tonsils, dental implants, the jawbones (cavitations), and the sinuses, along with any associated soft tissue infections and infections in the draining lymphatic network.

Some groups... claim the "theory" that focal infection can seed and fuel chronic disease was disproven by researchers over 80 years ago. Not so!

Along with the many clinical observations made by countless physicians and dentists over the last hundred years, there is substantial mainstream documentation in the scientific literature supporting a primary causal link between oral sites of chronic infection and a majority of man's most debilitating and life-threatening diseases.

Some groups like the American Dental Association and the American Association of Endodontists claim the "theory" that focal infection can seed and fuel chronic disease was disproven by researchers over 80 years ago. Not so! Even a cursory look at the peer-reviewed medical literature of the last 20 years shows the exact opposite conclusion to be true. Unfortunately, in spite of volumes of recent documentation affirming the links between focal infection and chronic disease, the truth has been effectively ignored and even discounted as having little or only trivial relevance in today's practice of medicine and dentistry.

This chapter demonstrates the now indisputable cause-and-effect relationship between focal infection, specifically in the teeth and gums, and some chronic diseases such as coronary artery disease. Until recently, the etiological links between oral infections and diseases, such as heart disease, cancer, and neurological disorders, were powerfully implicated but could not be proven. For decades, the lack of "smoking gun" evidence has provided cover for those who needed to "debunk" such evidence, claiming associations and correlations but nothing more. But now there is no place for denial. Modern and very sophisticated forms of testing have confirmed cause-and-effect connections—beyond a shadow of any doubt.

Statistically speaking...very few individuals with one or more chronic degenerative diseases, especially heart disease and cancer, are completely free from at least one significant oral cavity site of infection.

Statistically speaking, it will be shown that very few individuals with one or more chronic degenerative diseases, especially heart disease and cancer, are completely free from at least one significant oral cavity site of infection.

Furthermore, such infections are silent and typically remain undiagnosed. Finally, it will be shown that the inability to identify and/or eradicate such a site of infection remains the major obstacle to stopping the progression of such a chronic disease, or to even possibly reversing or resolving it.

Infected Teeth
Root Canal-Treated Teeth

In Chapter 3 we presented studies that demonstrate the ***cause-and-effect*** relationship between root canal-treated teeth and chronic disease. Some of those investigations tied root canal-treated teeth to the formation of the blood clots that block blood flow in the coronary arteries and cause myocardial infarctions. Other studies showed connections from these treated teeth to other degenerative processes. The bottom line is:

> **Root canal-treated teeth are the direct cause for the vast majority of heart attacks, period.**

And although all root canal-treated teeth have the potential for causing a host of diseases and conditions (in addition to heart disease), not all root canal-treated teeth pose the same degree of health risk. This reality starts with the procedure itself. From the outset, the "success" of a root canal procedure is highly variable. It usually depends primarily upon the experience and expertise of the dentist performing the procedure.

One marker of this success can be determined by a examining a post-procedure X-ray for apical radiolucency, or dark space around one or more root tips. Certain tissues, like bone, teeth, and cartilage are radiopaque, meaning that X-ray photons do not pass through them and therefore leave a "white" shadow on the X-ray. Areas filled with infection are radiolucent because some of the bony structure in the jaw has been resorbed, and the photons easily pass through them and leave an exposed (dark) spot on the X-ray (see examples in Appendix D). Therefore, a radiolucent (dark) area around the tip of a tooth indicates infection, called chronic apical periodontitis (CAP). A radiopaque (white) area indicates healthy tissue and bone surrounding the tooth's root tips.

> *Although all root canal-treated teeth have the potential for causing a host of diseases and conditions, not all root canal-treated teeth pose the same degree of health risk.*

Without a doubt, a root canal-treated tooth that demonstrates this degree of "success" (no radiolucency around the tooth root) after a root canal procedure is preferable to an untreated tooth with X-ray evidence of CAP. This is because a root canal-treated tooth without CAP will produce a substantially less long-term pathogen/toxin exposure than an untreated tooth with CAP. And, this is especially true when there is no gradual recurrence of CAP in the root canal-treated tooth on follow-up examinations.

In other words, we can roughly rate the severity of health risk from infected teeth as follows:

1. Normal tooth free of infection (no risk)
2. Root canal-treated tooth free of CAP (moderate risk)
3. Untreated tooth with CAP (great to severe risk)
4. Root canal-treated tooth with CAP (severe risk), especially when the CAP is recurring after initial resolution or near-resolution post-procedure

The tooth pain/ sensitivity that caused a patient to seek dental care indicates that serious problems are already brewing.

Before a root canal procedure is performed, however, the tooth pain/sensitivity that caused a patient to seek dental care indicates that serious problems are already brewing. Much more often than not, when a tooth is painful, it is already infected, and the pulp of the tooth is already necrotic and technically dead.

The purported goal of a root canal treatment is to rout out the infected, necrotic core (pulp) of the tooth, put in a sealant to prevent further chronic seeding of infection down into the apices (root tips), and render the tooth sterile. This goal of sterility is never completely achievable.

However, many individuals appear to do well when the periapical infection is largely removed, and no significant CAP remains or recurs.

The reason that a root canal procedure can never achieve a sterile outcome is that it is a "fatally-flawed" procedure...

Admittedly, a technically well-performed root canal procedure can "debulk" the amount of infection present and make it less prone to aggressive dissemination into the lymphatic and venous drainage of the jawbone. And that's certainly preferable to doing nothing and allowing the infected tooth to remain. A healthy tooth is internally sterile, but once infected, it will never be free of infecting pathogens again. This is true even if it is not grossly abscessed or demonstrating infectious apical pathology readily detectable on X-ray examination.

In fact, the reason that a root canal procedure can never achieve a sterile outcome is that it is a "fatally-flawed" procedure, at least with regard to completely curing any infection that is present. The practical impact of the procedure, as noted above, is to eliminate and evacuate as much of the pulp of the tooth as possible, and to seal it well enough to prevent continuous infectious leakage into the apical areas.

When the pulp has been largely removed, the immune system no longer has a way to reach the pathogens that remain in the miles (up to two or more miles in a single tooth) of dentinal tubules that radiate away from the pulp of the tooth. Immune cells need a physical framework to get from point A to point B. When the pulp, with its rich innervation, blood supply, and connective tissue structural components, is gone, the immune system loses the physical ability to reach the infected dentinal tubules with any efficacy whatsoever.

Additionally, the removal of all the nerves in the pulp disables and often destroys the tooth's disease detection system...

Additionally, the removal of all the nerves in the pulp disables and often destroys the tooth's disease detection system, the very system that created the pain for which the patient was seeking treatment. Typically, this absence of pain, especially if the patient is comfortable chewing normally, is usually the sole measure of the procedure's success, at least as far as the patient is concerned. Unfortunately, the lack of pain says absolutely nothing about the actual clinical status of the tooth since the nerves that signal the presence of infection have been removed or severed.

Furthermore, even in the rarest of circumstances when the pulp was not infected (probably misdiagnosed) prior to the root canal procedure, the removal of the pulp assures that the tooth will become and then forever remain infected. Pathogens normally colonizing the mouth have no problem entering the dentinal tubules and the treated/evacuated pulp space after a root canal procedure is performed. So, even though the tooth that has been "successfully" treated with a root canal procedure might remain pain-free, it remains chronically infected and a source of chronic toxin production for as long as it remains in the mouth.

As if that were not enough of a problem, the root canal-treated tooth is the perfect endogenous pathogen/toxin delivery system. Even though the pulp has been removed, the venous and lymphatic drainage of the bony socket holding the tooth remains intact. Every time the treated tooth is involved in chewing, the enormous pressures generated by this activity effectively squeeze accumulating pathogens and toxins directly into the lymphatic and venous systems of the jawbone and then throughout the body. Every chewing motion

> *The root canal-treated tooth is the perfect endogenous pathogen/toxin delivery system.*

covertly injects pathogens and toxins into the circu-latory/lymphatic systems just as efficiently as a syringe used to administer medicines to a sleeping patient.

The proof that a root canal-treated tooth can never result in a sterile tooth free of pathogens comes from the work of Dr. Boyd Haley of the University of Kentucky. Dr. Haley, initially in collabora-tion with Dr. Hal Huggins and later with a network of dentists around the country, tested over 5,000 consecutive extracted root canal-treated teeth.

While...some extracted root canal-treated teeth demonstrated decidedly more toxicity than others, significant toxicity was nevertheless found in 100% of these teeth.

Dr. Haley developed a process called nucleotide photo affinity labeling in order to see how effectively the toxins eluted from such teeth would inhibit the activity of five different human enzymes involved in the production of energy in the body (phosphor-ylase kinase, phosphorylase A, pyruvate kinase, creatine kinase, and adenylate kinase). The toxins that Dr. Haley found in these teeth were so concen-trated that the toxic impact of the different teeth could not be measured effectively in a comparative fashion until the third "washing" of the tooth suffi-ciently diluted the toxin presence.

While Dr. Haley did find that some extracted root canal-treated teeth demonstrated decidedly more toxicity than others, significant toxicity was nevertheless found in 100% of these teeth. Normal teeth extracted for orthodontic purposes demonstrated no measurable toxicity, ruling out the notion that some sort of oral cavity contamination of the extracted teeth resulted in the measured toxicity. The conclusion is clear: the root canal procedure, because of the mechanisms discussed above, always results in a toxic and chronically infected tooth.[1]

The microbial flora of primary root canal infections is a bit staggering in scope. Fungi, viruses, and over 460 different types of bacteria have been identified and reported in untreated primary root canal infections as well as in root canal-treated teeth.[2-4] Sometimes the bacteria found in these infections are not even felt to be related to the usual microflora of the mouth.[5] Generally, the endodontic literature only examines the pathogen content of "failed" root canal-treated teeth that demonstrate persistent significant CAP and/or continue to be painful. However, as all such teeth are chronically infected, it can be readily appreciated that the flora reported in such studies would

The root canal procedure, because of the mechanisms discussed above, always results in a toxic and chronically infected tooth.

be the same as for teeth that were treated "success-fully," except that the "failed" root canal-treated tooth is symptomatic. These teeth may or may not show X-ray evidence of CAP, although 3D cone beam imaging will detect this finding to some degree the vast majority of the time.

While the evidence is clear that all root canal-treated teeth are infected, it is also clear that the negative clinical impact of one or more such teeth on the general health is highly variable.

Other studies have looked at the endotoxins found in root canal-treated teeth. Endotoxins are toxins produced by certain gram-negative bacteria that reside on the outer membrane and can inde-pendently produce negative health impacts aside from those initiated by the presence of the pathogen itself. Of the teeth tested in two different studies, 100% produced detectable endotoxins. One study detected the endotoxins in 21 out of 21 teeth, and the other study detected endo-toxins in 30 out of 30 teeth.[6,7]

While the evidence is clear that all root canal-treated teeth are infected, it is also clear that the negative clinical impact of one or more such teeth on the general health is highly variable. Without a doubt, there are some 90-year-old persons who have had such teeth for decades, feel great, and have normal routine laboratory test results, including

C-reactive protein. In addition to typically having especially strong immune systems, such individuals also usually have normal thyroid and sex hormone status, or they have been receiving optimal hormone replacement therapy. On the other side of the spectrum, there are those 55-year-old individuals who undergo a single root canal procedure and then sustain a heart attack a few months later.

Nobody's clinical circumstances are alike. What can kill one person quickly may have no discernible effect on another. Whether or not an infected tooth has been treated, multiple factors can play a role in the severity of clinical impact that an infected tooth can inflict on a given patient. These include the following:

✓ The unique pathogen flora present, including bacteria, viruses, fungi, and protozoa, and their unique interactions (infection-related mediators, enzymes, and production of other infection-spreading agents) and even synergistic toxic impact[8-13]

✓ The tooth involved (small incisor versus large molar: an incisor with smaller quantity of infection is much less critical than a molar with greater quantity of infection and much greater capacity to disseminate that infection upon chewing)

✓ Infection containment (the degree to which the bone surrounding the socket becomes cavitated, further facilitating dissemination; or whether the CAP is largely uncontained or more effectively contained by the formation of a chronic fibrous encapsulation)

✓ Genetic predisposition to different diseases

✓ How long the tooth has been infected or has had the root canal procedure

✓ The quality of digestion and nutrition

✓ The quantity and quality of vitamins, minerals, and other nutrient supplements taken regularly

✓ Hormonal status (sex hormones and especially thyroid which directly and strongly affect the likelihood and degree to which pathogens can disseminate and take hold remotely—as in the coronary and cerebral artery endothelial layers, and in the breasts in women via connecting lymphatic channels)

✓ Age, general health, and bone health of the patient (significant jawbone osteopenia; immunocompetence; compromise of jawbone health post-radiotherapy)[14]

Teeth with Radiographic Apical Lesions

An apical lesion on X-ray typically refers to a radiolucency at the tip of one or more root tips of the affected tooth. This radiographic lesion is known as apical periodontitis, and when it has been documented to be present for an extended period of time, it is known as chronic apical periodontitis (CAP). Whether acute or chronic, this X-ray finding means that, in addition to being infected, the root canal system or pulp of the tooth is dead and has precipitated a significant flow of pathogens into the area surrounding the root tips. This egress of pathogens results in a spectrum of pathologies in addition to the immune response generated by presence of those pathogens. These range from a bone-resorbing, pus-filled abscess to a fibrotic granuloma, or even a cyst.[15-17]

Regardless of the particular pathogens identified after extraction, all X-ray pictures of CAP are largely the same, and the negative clinical consequences are essentially the same as well. In other words, there are several common situations that will generate an X-ray picture of apical periodontitis (radiolucency).

Even though the X-ray appearance is the same, and the negative health impacts are largely identical, the specific dental/clinical approach to remediation of these infections is far from uniform. As a practical point, the chosen method of treatment is determined when dentist preferences, patient preferences, and potential acute and long-term health impact on the patient are factored together. Common clinical conditions and typical treatments, while NOT necessarily being recommended, include the following:

- ✓ **Painful acute apical periodontitis**. Usually exquisitely painful and palpably tender due to an abscess at the tip of one or more roots of a tooth, this infection seems to manifest suddenly. Typical clinical approaches range from immediate extraction with thorough cleaning of the bony socket to apical abscess drainage (apicoectomy). This drainage is usually followed with a root canal procedure. Both approaches would also involve a course of antibiotics and various ozone applications, if available, for treatment of infection and prevention of its spread.
- ✓ **Symptomatic chronic apical periodontitis (CAP)**. This refers to the tooth that does not become acutely and overwhelming painful but instead can be intermittently minimally to moderately painful with discomfort on chewing over an extended period of time. The approach to this tooth would be much the same as above, except there would usually be no need for the apicoectomy. Antibiotics and

ozone treatments would be indicated as well.

✓ **Asymptomatic chronic apical periodontitis (CAP)**. Far and away, this is the most common presentation of an infected tooth that has not been given a prior root canal procedure. Ironically, the pain-free CAP tooth represents a source of pathogens and toxins that have a much greater negative clinical impact than is already seen with a root canal-treated tooth that has little to no residual apical pathology on X-ray. Extraction allow, root canal treatment, or extraction immediately followed by an implant would be the main options. Infection resolution measures, such as ozone and antibiotics, would always be indicated as well.

✓ **Post-root canal treatment of chronic apical periodontitis (CAP)**. Many of the teeth that receive root canal treatments initially present with at least some degree of CAP, along with pain. The technical success of the root canal procedure is generally measured in terms of pain relief and the absence or significant lessening in size of the apical radiolucencies on X-ray. When CAP later reappears, or begins to enlarge, the root canal-treated tooth is considered to have recurrent apical pathology and active infection.

As with the above categories of tooth infection, extraction or a repeat root canal procedure are the usual approaches, although a repeat procedure is really never a good option when the first procedure failed.

Untreated teeth with CAP, even when asymptomatic (which is **_usually_** the case), are **_highly_** toxic. They can substantially contribute to the initiation and provocation of multiple chronic degenerative diseases, especially heart disease and breast cancer. A CAP infection is often part of the reason for performing a root canal procedure. Consequently, the array of toxins and pathogens that are seen in a CAP tooth are also present in the root canal-treated tooth. The only major difference is that these toxins and pathogens are present in greater volume in the CAP tooth since the infection has not been debulked with the pulp chamber effectively sealed off by an **optimally** performed root canal procedure.

> *Consequently, the array of toxins and pathogens that are seen in a CAP tooth are also present in the root canal-treated tooth.*

It is important to note that even a well-performed root canal procedure never **_eliminates_** infection and toxicity. However, when CAP disappears or is minimized post-procedure and ***does not recur***, it is likely that the procedure has significantly lessened the pathogen/toxin impact on the body. The quality of the apical seal following a root canal procedure would appear to be the primary factor in eliminating or lessening infectious microleakage from the treated tooth into the apical areas, resulting in the presence or worsening of CAP.[18]

This was demonstrated quite impressively in a study that estimated the atherosclerotic burden in the abdominal aorta using a calcium scoring method. In a total of 11,191 teeth examined by computed tomography in 531 patients, the atherosclerotic burden increased when more CAP teeth were present that did not receive root canal treatments. However, in patients who had root canal-treated teeth with some CAP no consistent correlation to atherosclerotic burden was found. This further indicates the benefit of infection debulking by the root canal procedure when extraction was not considered to be an option.[19]

The greater the endodontic burden, the greater the chances of heart attack, angina, or heart-related death.

It has already shown epidemiologically that the very presence of any root canal-treated tooth, with no further qualification, is related to an increased risk of coronary heart disease. Therefore, the lack of correlation reported in the study just cited cannot be used to conclude that root canal-treated teeth are completely safe. It only shows that they are generally less toxic than untreated CAP teeth.

Another more recent study found that CAP produced a 5.3 fold increase of cardiovascular disease risk compared to patients without CAP.

The total negative health impact of CAP teeth and root canal-treated teeth, termed the "endodontic burden" was examined in another study. The greater the endodontic burden, the greater the chances of heart attack, angina, or heart-related death.[20] Another group came to similar conclusions when examining the negative impact of CAP of various degrees of severity, with and without previous root canal treatments.[21] Others have demonstrated that there is a direct correlation between the actual size (calculated volume) of CAP radiolucencies and the quantities of endotoxins produced by the infection.[22]

In two studies that attempted to quantify the increased risk of cardiovascular disease associated with CAP, the results were striking. In one study, coronary angiography demonstrated that patients with CAP had a 2.79 times higher risk of developing coronary artery disease.[23] Another more recent study found that CAP produced a 5.3 fold increase of cardiovascular disease risk compared to patients without CAP.[24] The results of the first study are impressive, but the findings of the second study are quite stunning.

Another investigation also documented this clear association between CAP and cardiovascular disease.[25] Cumulatively, these studies loudly affirm the following conclusion:

> **CAP of any degree, even if completely silent, pain-free, and only incidentally discovered on X-ray, should never be ignored.**

Quite the contrary, there should always be an ***active effort*** to identify this radiographic entity in the workup of any patient with one or more chronic degenerative diseases—especially heart disease and breast cancer. Although extraction is not the only therapeutic option for such a tooth, it is always the best option when the long-term

There is already clear-cut documentation that root canal-treated teeth directly cause the majority of heart attacks

cardiac and general health of the patient is the overriding concern. Ironically, on a internet blog that receives a lot of visits from dentists, the high incidence of asymptomatic CAP detected on 3D cone beam imaging has some dentists wondering what to do and whether such teeth should just be ignored. The answer, however, is simple. Never leave such teeth unaddressed when the general health of the patient is of primary concern.

Since there is already clear-cut documentation that root canal-treated teeth directly cause the majority of heart attacks, the study cited above takes on even greater significance.[19] The following can now be asserted, based on this study and the earlier work demonstrating the high concentration of root canal pathogens in the blood clots causing myocardial infarctions:[26]

> Asymptomatic, pain-free teeth with the X-ray findings of chronic apical periodontitis (CAP) will be expected to have an ***even greater negative*** impact on coronary atherosclerosis and on chronic degenerative diseases than the root canal-treated tooth, with or without associated CAP.

> Additionally, since all of these infected teeth contain the same pathogenic bacteria, ***any study linking a disease or medical condition to any form of chronic periodontitis also effectively links CAP and/or the root canal-treated tooth to the same condition***.

Infected Gums and Tooth Supportive Tissue (General Periodontitis)

Periodontal disease can range from inflammation of the most superficial aspects of the gum tissue (gingivitis) to the chronic inflammation and loss of tooth-supporting tissues (advanced periodontitis), including bone.[27] General periodontitis, or periodontal disease, starts as an infectious condition of the gum tissue directly surrounding the tooth that can eventually involve the bone supporting the tooth. When left unchecked, this can further evolve to its most advanced form, chronic apical periodontitis (CAP), with potential tooth loss a possibility.

Initially, bacteria proliferate on the gingiva and in the space between the superficial gum surfaces and the tooth known as the sulcus. This gingivitis leads directly to periodontitis when the enzymes produced by the more common periodontal pathogens cause damage to the gingival tissues that progress into the tooth root and supporting bone, progressively separating the tooth root from the tissue surrounding the tooth and working down to the surrounding jawbone, much like unzipping a zipper. This results in bone resorption, visible as darker areas or radiolucencies on X-ray.

The degree of periodontal infection can be reliably estimated by looking at the depth of the radiolucency between the tooth and bony socket, along with how deeply these areas can be probed on dental examination. CAP can ultimately result when the pathogens advance all the way down the side of the tooth to the root tips and begin to resorb the surrounding jawbone to produce its classical X-ray picture of an apical dark space. CAP can also result from infection of the tooth pulp from above, as with deep caries that breach the tooth pulp. Nevertheless, the pathogen/toxin profile, X-ray appearance, and clinical impact of the resulting CAP picture are the same.

Arguably, CAP represents the single most important cause of chronic disease that can be addressed and eliminated.

As discussed more thoroughly in Chapter 1, the major difference between general periodontitis and CAP is the severity of the infection since both are chronic infections that share virtually identical pathogen profiles, and both elevate inflammatory biomarkers of oxidative stress throughout the body.[28]

It bears repeating that at the very minimum any condition linked to general periodontitis can also be attributed to any tooth with CAP, which is the most advanced form of periodontitis. Therefore, periodontitis of any kind needs immediate attention and remediation.

How Common is Chronic Apical Periodontitis (CAP)?

While variably present in different populations (for specific statistics see Chapter 1), CAP is nevertheless very common, particularly in a ***painless, asymptomatic*** state. Yet, any CAP tooth can be expected to negatively impact the general health, and oftentimes ***it can be the primary reason why someone has a heart attack or contracts cancer***. Arguably, CAP represents the single most important cause of chronic disease that can be addressed and eliminated. Sometimes, after proper tooth removal and with the provision of optimal dietary, supplemental, and hormonal support, patients experience the actual reversal of what is traditionally considered irreversible disease. Anybody with any chronic degenerative disease, especially heart disease and cancer, needs to have an oral pathology evaluation as part of the routine initial medical evaluation. Any oral pathology,

3D cone beam computed tomography has brought resolution to a new level, and pathology is now often detected when it is not seen on regular X-rays.

especially asymptomatic CAP, needs to be appropriately treated. Otherwise, the patient's best chance for health improvement has been forfeited. And the best chance for preventing serious health problems in the future has been lost as well. New cancers or cancer recurrences will often result after initially "successful" cancer treatments when CAP teeth are ignored.

A very important factor in determining the true prevalence of CAP depends upon the quality of the diagnostic examination. Most studies still report on the incidence of apical pathology based on full-mouth X-rays (panoramic radiographs). Focal periapical radiographs, especially with digital subtraction technology, improve detail substantially.[29,30] But most recently 3D cone beam computed tomography has brought resolution to a new level (see Appendix D for examples), and pathology is now often detected when it is not seen on regular X-rays.[31]

It is likely that 3D examination is consistently at least 40% and perhaps even 50% better in finding periapical pathology than using a standard panoramic X-ray.

In a study that directly compared the X-ray examination of 46 root canal-treated teeth with the 3D cone beam CT examination of the **_same_** teeth, CAP was found in 32 of 46 teeth (70%) by intraoral X-ray. The 3D technology found CAP in 42 of the 46 teeth (91%). Three oral radiologists examined all of the images.[32]

Furthermore, intraoral X-ray produces significantly improved images compared to standard panoramic X-rays. Such panoramic X-ray studies are the type of X-ray that was used for nearly all of the CAP prevalence studies itemized in Chapter 1. It has been shown that 3D examinations find periapical pathology roughly 30% more often than intraoral X-ray.[33,34] Another study showed that the 3D technology found apical lesions more than twice as often as digital radiography [35% of the teeth studied versus 14%].[35] It is likely that 3D examination is consistently at least 40% and perhaps even 50% better in finding periapical pathology than using a standard panoramic X-ray.[36-39]

Furthermore, histopathological studies in dog teeth indicate that even 3D examination misses a small percent of apical pathology.[40]

In reviewing the statistics on CAP, it is now apparent that the presence of asymptomatic CAP discoverable only by X-ray or cone beam imaging is extremely common. This means that at least one such tooth is likely present in a majority of adults around the world today, generally increasing in both prevalence and incidence with increasing age. This is not surprising, as older individuals have more chronic

> *Of the total abutment teeth that were not root-filled, 25% had associated CAP. Of the abutment teeth that were root canal-treated, 47% had associated CAP.*

disease. Depending upon the study and the population being examined, the prevalence of asymptomatic CAP in **_untreated_** teeth ranged between 0.8% to 9% in studies utilizing regular X-ray examinations. Considering that these numbers were generated with "regular" X-ray examinations, this means than 3D examination of the same untreated teeth could be expected to reveal CAP pathology roughly between 1.2% and 13.5% of the time.

> *CAP is the main cause and aggravator of heart disease, cancer, and most chronic diseases.*

To further underscore the high prevalence of CAP in asymptomatic teeth, there is another subset of teeth that demonstrate CAP on X-ray a very high percentage of the time. Abutment teeth, the teeth that are used to support or anchor crowns and bridges, were specifically examined in one study. A total of 4,656 abutment teeth out of 22,280 teeth on 1,000 patients were identified and reviewed. Of the total abutment teeth that were not root-filled, 25% had associated CAP. Of the abutment teeth that were root canal-treated, 47% had associated CAP.[40] Only regular X-rays were reviewed in this study, so it could be anticipated that 3D cone beam examination would probably find CAP in 30% to 35% of the untreated abutment teeth and in 65% to 75% of the root-filled abutment teeth. But even without this extrapolation, the number of abutment teeth that are chronically infected is still very high, and particular attention should be paid to the thorough and complete examination of these teeth in patients with heart disease and other significant chronic degenerative diseases.

To recap, 3D examination finds some degree of CAP in as many as 90% of root canal-treated teeth. Add to that the fact that 50% to 80% of most adult populations around the world have at least one root canal-treated tooth (based on studies cited earlier). Then add to that the high incidence of CAP in untreated teeth. And along with all of that consider the mounds of evidence presented in Chapter 3 that links periodontitis to chronic disease. At this juncture the following conclusion is inescapable:

> ***CAP** is **the** **main** **cause** **and** **aggravator** **of** **heart** **disease,** **cancer,** **and** **most** **chronic** **diseases***. Unfortunately this pandemic infection, whether in a root-filled tooth or an untreated tooth, is rarely diagnosed and almost never properly addressed.

CAP is highly toxic whether it is present with an untreated, asymptomatic tooth or with a tooth that has previously received a root canal treatment. Any evidence of infection in a tooth needs to be regarded as having a negative impact on health, oftentimes to a life-threatening degree. Nevertheless, some infected teeth are much more noxious than others.

The following is a listing of different infected tooth scenarios, very roughly from the most toxic scenario to the least toxic scenario.

1. The very painful, acutely abscessed tooth with a large CAP lesion, untreated
2. The asymptomatic to mildly symptomatic tooth with a large CAP lesion, untreated
3. The asymptomatic to mildly symptomatic tooth with large CAP lesion, root-filled
4. The asymptomatic to mildly symptomatic tooth with small CAP lesion, untreated
5. The asymptomatic tooth, root-filled, with continued significant CAP following the procedure, toxicity depending on the size of the lesion
6. The asymptomatic to mildly symptomatic tooth with small CAP lesion, root-filled; relatively lower toxicity when the lesion has decreased following the root canal treatment versus no change in the size of the lesion; relatively higher toxicity when the lesion has increased in size after the root canal treatment
7. The asymptomatic to mildly symptomatic tooth with evidence of only apical inflammation, with minimal widening of the space between the tooth root and the

periodontal ligament on X-ray (a potential precursor to the later development
of CAP)

8. The asymptomatic root canal-treated
tooth without any CAP, or with resolution of pre-existing CAP and no evidence
of recurrence for six months or more

9. The ***properly*** extracted untreated tooth
or root canal-treated tooth with CAP
lesion; of note, poor infection/toxin
protection and improper technique in
extracting an infected tooth can result in
myocardial infarction[42,43]

10. The dental implant after complete
healing has taken place, depending
on whether minimal, moderate, or
advanced peri-implantitis is present

Other factors that affect the degree of toxic
impact that an infected tooth has on the general
health include hormonal balance (mainly thyroid
and sex hormone),[44] and the quality of pre-existing
general health and immunocompetence. Another
measure of the health impact appears in laboratory
parameters that track body-wide inflammation and
infection, such as C-reactive protein and cytokine
levels, both systemically and inside the CAP lesions
themselves.[45-49]

The Histopathology of Chronic Apical Periodontitis (CAP)

CAP evolves from an inflammatory reaction to pathogens that have infected the root canal system (pulp) of the tooth, resulting in the necrosis or death of the pulp. Subsequently, pathogens colonize the root canal space. Eventually, these pathogens and their toxic metabolic byproducts seep through one or more roots and seed and colonize the areas surrounding the tooth root tips (apical areas), usually growing over time. The initial pulp infection typically results from caries, trauma, or excessive dental intervention that breaches the pulp space (which normally should be sterile), and the oral microbial flora gains access. Sometimes the primary infection comes from advanced periodontitis eventually reaching and colonizing the root tips, and then the root canal system becomes necrotic and chronically infected in a retrograde fashion from the root tips upward. This the less common scenario.

Whether the infection starts in the tooth or in the surrounding tissues, the X-ray of the CAP tooth looks the same and the root canal system of the affected tooth is always necrotic and chronically infected. Although an X-ray picture reliably shows the presence of a significant apical infection, it cannot provide any details concerning the pathological reactions of the affected tissues. For that reason, the clinical impact of CAP on the body and general health is quite variable. And although infection is the common underlying cause, the way in which the body and immune defenses react to that infection largely determine the toxicity of the CAP tooth, much like the root canal-treated tooth.

Evidence for infection always being the cause of CAP is further demonstrated in a compelling animal study in which tooth pulps were exposed to the oral cavity in experimentally germ-free rats, resulting in no CAP, while control rats with typical oral micro-flora developed massive apical radiolucencies as the infection took hold in those exposed pulps.[50]

Factors that impact and determine the clinical toxicity of a CAP tooth include the following:

✓ The intrinsic virulence of the infecting/ colonizing pathogens, including the production of endotoxins and infection-spreading proteolytic enzymes[51]

✓ The combined/synergistic virulence of multiple microbes/pathogens[52,53]

✓ The strength and competence of the patient's immune system and other defense mechanisms

✓ The underlying histopathology of the periapical lesion (infection with acute abscess formation, infection with granuloma formation, walled off by

connective tissue, and infection with the
development of an encapsulating apical
cyst)

These different factors determining the clinical
impact of CAP are mentioned to highlight that one
X-ray appearance is consistent with a number of
different underlying pathophysiological processes.
Furthermore, it is the first three factors mentioned
above that will largely determine the degree of
negative clinical impact, along with the age of the
periapical lesion, and whether the X-ray represents
an abscess, granuloma, or cyst. One study of 256
lesions examined upon extraction showed 35% to
be abscesses, 50% to be granulomas, and 15% to be
cysts.[54] However, all of the pathologies are toxic, and
it is always best to properly remove such a tooth,
since the pulp of the tooth is infected and necrotic
(dead), and it will always be a steady endogenous
source of significant toxins, and even possibly a
source of pathogens that can seed and take hold
elsewhere in the body.

Conclusion

Oral cavity infections, especially infected
teeth and gums, are the most important factors
that consistently and profoundly exert negative
impact on the general health today. Infected teeth
have been shown to be extremely common in the
adult populations throughout the world, and they

primarily take the form of root canal-treated teeth, along with other teeth, usually painless, that have not been root canal-treated but are in chronic states of infection (teeth with chronic apical periodontitis [CAP]). Root canal-treated teeth also very commonly have some degree of CAP associated with them. All CAP teeth, whether untreated or following root canal procedures, need to be tracked carefully for the rest of the life of the patient, along with CRP blood testing. The best follow-up will utilize repeated 3D cone beam imaging.

Advanced infected gum disease, or chronic periodontitis, has long been strongly linked to nearly all chronic degenerative diseases that have been studied with regard to this association. CAP is the most advanced form of chronic periodontitis, meaning it shares all of the disease associations reported with less advanced forms of gum infection.

A cause-and-effect relationship between heart attacks and the pathogens found in root canal-treated teeth and chronic periodontitis has now been established. These same pathogens are found in the chronically infected, yet asymptomatic CAP teeth. This means that infected teeth with CAP also directly cause atherosclerosis and heart attacks, and it is likely, although not equally proven at this point, that this cause-and-effect relationship exists between CAP and very many, likely most, of the other chronic degenerative diseases. Increasing evidence is now allowing the reasonable conclusion that infected teeth and gums are the most common cause of breast cancer.

As multiple studies have clearly demonstrated that the asymptomatic CAP tooth is a very common entity, the optimal medical evaluation and management of all patients with chronic degenerative diseases, especially heart disease and cancer, must include 3D cone beam imaging of all of the teeth, as a baseline and in periodic follow-up examinations, along with regular blood testing, especially of CRP levels. When such teeth are present and remain unidentified and unextracted, the best chance for disease improvement and even disease resolution remains forever missed.

Infected Tonsils

Overview

Of all oral infections chronic apical periodontitis (CAP), in both treated and untreated teeth, mounts the most dangerous and consequential assault against good health. However, asymptomatic, infected palatine tonsils (tonsils) also have an ominous potential to initiate and promote body-wide disease, especially in the adult population. Prior to passing the point of no return, tonsils usually offer a minimal degree of immune protection against common oropharyngeal infections or pathogen colonizations. However, as will be demonstrated, they are easily overwhelmed by more severe chronic oral infections, such as CAP, root canal-treated teeth, and even general periodontitis. These pathogen sources cause the tonsils to become chronically and irreversibly infected. At that point they cease to protect against disease but rather promote it.

Pathophysiology

What is not in dispute, however, is that the tonsils of many individuals eventually become chronically infected and negatively impact health.

Palatine tonsils are the two dense bodies of lymphoid tissue located in the back of the mouth, one on each side of the throat. As part of their immune function, they produce immunoglobulins and exert lymphocyte-mediated immune responses, including antibody production from B cells and cell-mediated immune responses from T cells.[1]

Nevertheless, for a variety of reasons, a substantial amount of debate continues over how clinically important the tonsils are in defending the individual against pathogens. What is not in dispute, however, is that the tonsils of many individuals eventually become chronically infected and negatively impact health. Any tonsil with a chronic, non-resolving infection or abscess can readily disseminate pathogens and pathogen-related toxins throughout the body via tonsillar drainage into the venous and lymphatic systems.

Visual examination of tonsils, especially those that have experienced recurrent tonsillitis, often leaves no question that they are chronically infected. However, a very large number of chronically infected tonsils, even when the infection is severe, maintain a normal external appearance.

A microscopic study of the tonsil reveals that there are many invaginations of the external surface of the tonsils known as crypts. These crypts greatly increase the surface area of the tonsillar tissue, presumably to increase a tonsil's ability to intercept and immunologically process a larger amount of pathogens. However, when the ability of the tonsil to process pathogens becomes chronically overwhelmed, it seems that these same crypts become reservoirs for pathogens and their metabolic byproducts. When this occurs, non-resolving pockets of pus (abscesses) often form within the crypts and even on the tonsillar surface.

...a very large number of chronically infected tonsils, even when the infection is severe, maintain a normal external appearance.

In general, the tonsils are suitable for processing smaller pathogen challenges on an intermittent basis, rather than larger, continuous pathogen assaults.

Why Tonsils Become Chronically Infected

Any root canal-treated tooth or any tooth displaying chronic apical periodontitis (CAP) upon

X-ray examination exposes the draining tonsil to an enormous and continual source of pathogens and pathogen-related toxins. While it is likely that both tonsils offer some drainage to one side of the jawbone, the same-side (ipsilateral) tonsil will have to "filter" a fairly constant stream of pathogens as long as the chronically infected tooth remains in the mouth. This intimate pathway between the tonsils and the teeth has been elegantly demonstrated by injecting Indian ink into a sealed dental cavity. Within 20 to 30 minutes of the injections, ink spots will appear on the tonsillar surface. Chronically infected gum tissue (chronic periodontitis) also displays this intimate connection with the lymphatic drainage network of the tonsils. Indian ink rubbed onto the gums similarly appears on the tonsils in short order.

This intimate pathway between the tonsils and the teeth has been elegantly demonstrated...

Over time, as a draining tonsil becomes more inflamed and chronically infected, the lymph flow through the tonsil tends to stagnate. Consequently, the restricted mouth-to-tonsil lymph flow that results pushes the excess lymphatic drainage from the gums and jawbone through alternative lymphatic and even venous pathways. This overflow of pathogen and toxin-laden lymph can overload the draining neck and chest lymphatic pathways. Of especially great importance and concern, this pathogenic drainage sets the stage for malignant transformation in the breast tissue of women as well as other chronic disease pathologies.

In 1951, Josef Issels, MD, established the first European hospital for "incurable" cancer patients in Germany. Much of his work at this clinic is documented in his landmark book, *Cancer, A Second Opinion*. Many of the following observations on tonsillar pathology come from this work.[2]

This pathogenic drainage sets the stage for malignant transformation in the breast tissue of women as well as other chronic disease pathologies.

In a survey of the adult cancer patients that he saw at his clinic, Issels found that **98%** of them had between "two and ten dead teeth." Issels eventually incorporated routine tonsillectomy in his treatment protocol for these patients. Prior to instituting this practice he noted that roughly 40% of those whose did not survive died of a heart attack. This number dropped to 5% after tonsillectomy became routine. One of the more memorable observations of Issels, and there are many, was his following comment on tonsils:

> **Tonsils are the great curse of the body. They can appear normal. But on laboratory examination they are all found**

to be grossly infected in all cancer patients.

Considering the very high prevalence of infected teeth in his cancer patients, along with the fact that the tonsils continually provide the drainage for infected teeth and gums, the observations of Issels are of great value in appreciating the enormous negative impact that infected tonsils can have on the health status of the patient. Infected tonsils might well be the ultimate "Trojan horse" for harboring potent pathogens and toxins while appearing completely normal in routine oral examinations. Furthermore, it would appear that tonsils with advanced chronic infection can never be expected to heal, even after the offending infected teeth have been removed and/or the gum infections have resolved. Rather, they can undermine good health even _**decades**_ after the chronic oral infections have been removed or otherwise resolved.

> *Infected tonsils might well be the ultimate "Trojan horse" for harboring potent pathogens and toxins while appearing completely normal in routine oral examinations.*

Issels also made the following observations regarding the pathology of the tonsils that he routinely removed from his cancer patients:

> **The findings in these healthy-looking tonsils were incomparably more serious than even those in the obviously diseased tonsils removed in the usual ENT practice.**

> **...frequently there were several abscesses as well as cysts often the size of cherries, full of liquid or condensed pus. The tonsillar tissue was spongy, slushy, and had a putrid smell. Histological examination always showed severe degenerative changes, and in the majority of cases, a complete atrophy of lymphoepithelial tissue.**

Issels noted that he treated over 8,000 cancer patients during a period of 25 years. After he decided that tonsillectomy would always be included as part of his cancer treatment protocol for patients with chronically infected teeth, he made the following observation:

> **In *every* tonsillectomy performed in my clinic subsequently, we found through biopsy severe or very severe destructive tonsillar processes with more or less virulent tonsillogenic focal toxicosis.** (emphasis mine)

Anecdotally, my own personal experience with normal-appearing, but chronically infected tonsils mirrors the findings and clinical experiences of Issels. It also confirms the observation that a chronically infected and abscessed tonsil, even after a very long time, is unable to heal itself.

Several years ago I had the sudden onset of shortness of breath and chest tightness when I chased off a large, aggressive dog bent on attacking my small poodle. As a cardiologist, I instantly realized that this was a first-time occurrence of angina. And until it subsided about 5 to 10 minutes later, I had no idea whether it would proceed to a heart attack.

...I was certain that such consistent elevations of CRP indicated a state of chronic inflammation in my body.

I was 61 years of age at the time, and I had been very concerned for over 10 years with the abnormalities in my periodic blood testing. The results were consistent with those indicating metabolic syndrome. And this was in spite of doing everything I felt possible to improve those numbers.

Of even greater concern to me was the fact that, during that same period of time, I had been maintaining an elevated CRP (C-reactive protein) level averaging between 4.5 to 5 mg/L. Since the reference range for CRP is 0 to 3 mg/L, and the true normal levels are below 0.5 mg/L, I was certain that such consistent elevations of CRP indicated a state of chronic inflammation in my body. It was also likely that the inflammation was secondary to an area of focal infection that was persistent and not resolving. This meant that my chances of developing coronary heart disease and having an acute cardiac event were substantially high. And after having my episode of chest tightness as described above, I was very certain that the increased chance of heart attack was no longer theoretical but instead quite likely without a significant intervention.

Previously I had demonstrated to my satisfaction that I could significantly lower my CRP with a week's worth of daily 100-gram vitamin C infusions. But, it would quickly elevate again once I discontinued such an intensive intravenous protocol. This further underscored the limitations of quality supplementation when underlying infectious pathology remains unaddressed.

Some 25 or so years earlier I had received a root canal in one of my molars on the left side of my lower jaw.

Some 25 or so years earlier I had received a root canal in one of my molars on the left side of my lower jaw. It had remained in my mouth until I developed high blood pressure and had it extracted some 5 years or so later on the suggestion of my mentor, Dr. Hal Huggins. Even though the root canal-treated tooth had been gone for nearly 20 years, I nevertheless began to wonder whether the left-sided tonsil could be chronically infected. The work of Dr. Issels strongly implied that this would be the case.

After the episode of chest pain I promptly made the decision that my tonsils had to be removed, and soon. Nothing I had done over the years was lowering my CRP, and I was not about to have a heart attack wondering whether my tonsils were taking away my good health.

I found an ENT doctor who agreed to take out my tonsils after I convinced him that I was tired of having recurrent tonsillitis, even though I had never had tonsillitis a single time. Since surgeons rarely need a lot of encouragement or justification to operate, he readily agreed to take my tonsils out upon hearing my fabricated history. He did note on my oral cavity examination that the tonsils looked a little enlarged, but otherwise appeared completely normal in appearance.

Upon hearing this news, I immediately knew I had done the right thing in getting the tonsillectomy.

When I saw my surgeon again following the procedure, I asked him how everything went. He commented that everything went well, but that he was a little surprised to see pus easily express from the left tonsil when he grabbed it for removal. Upon hearing this news, I immediately knew I had done the right thing in getting the tonsillectomy.

As it turned out, I had the opportunity to have a rapid cardiac CAT scan with the intravenous injection of a venous contrast agent about 6 months later. One of the arteries had a 40 to 50% narrowing in it. As I never had another episode of chest discomfort after the tonsillectomy, I was quite convinced that this moderate arterial narrowing had been critically narrowed six months earlier, but had since had the opportunity to at least partially regress.

But after the extraction my long-standing elevated CRP finally dropped well into the reference laboratory range at 2.02.

To be sure, undergoing a tonsillectomy as an adult was about the worst experience of my life, but I am also sure that I would have eventually had a heart attack had I not undergone the procedure— probably sooner rather than later.

Interestingly, my CRP dropped significantly after the tonsillectomy, but not completely into the reference laboratory range. It was not until another year and a half elapsed that another tooth, one that had not been root canal-treated, began to hurt. Eventually, it was extracted and showed obvious infection at the apex.

How long had it been infected while still being asymptomatic? There is no way to know for sure, but after the extraction my long-standing elevated CRP finally dropped well into the reference laboratory range at 2.02. One very good possibility is that this tooth had been a classical asymptomatic CAP tooth for years that finally become symptomatic, which can happen at any time for a number of reasons.[3] I had never had the 3D cone beam imaging of my teeth at that point in time, so there is no way to know for sure if this had been the case. But the data that now exists connecting a painless CAP tooth having substantial negative impact on cardiac and general health perfectly fits my clinical picture.

As long as the infected tonsils are not causing frequent colds or sore throats, or are not causing problems with breathing or swallowing, they are generally not even considered as being important factors in a patient's arthritis, asthma, nephritis, heart disease, or other chronic degenerative disease.

The Tonsils as Focal Infections

A small minority of physicians has long considered infected tonsils to be a prototypical example of focal infection causing and/or aggravating many different diseases remote from the oral cavity. That said, however, the vast majority of today's physicians do not even consider the possibility of chronically infected tonsils as even playing a minor role in causing or aggravating any of the illnesses they see in their patients. The degree to which the pathology in tonsils is ignored today is underscored by the fact that many older children and adults are not even considered as candidates for tonsillectomy when they have had recurrent tonsillitis and the tonsils are obviously grossly infected on cursory examination. As long as the infected tonsils are not causing frequent colds or sore throats, or are not causing problems with breathing or swallowing, they are generally not even considered as being important factors in a patient's arthritis, asthma, nephritis, heart disease, or other chronic degenerative disease.

Furthermore, their removal can often be the only intervention that offers any real hope as to reversal or even resolution of a given chronic disease.

Much of the time, however, such infected tonsils are the ***primary*** causes for such diseases. Furthermore, their removal can often be the only intervention that offers any real hope as to reversal or even resolution of a given chronic disease. And while a tonsillectomy in an older individual is not a trivial surgery,[4] the removal of chronically infected tonsils will always be a major boost to the immune system and general health even if a dramatic reversal of a chronic disease is not seen. Of note, it is now appearing that intermittent ozone injections directly into the tonsils can often lessen their infectious/toxic impact. Until more controlled studies are done, it remains to be seen whether such an intervention can restore an infected tonsil to normal, and if so, how often such a result can be anticipated.

Patients with recurrent tonsillitis often have discernible surface pathology on the tonsils. However, very many normal-appearing tonsils are severely infected.

Almost universally, unless an ENT specialist is the one performing the exam, little attention is paid to the tonsils during the routine physical examination. Most internists and general practitioners do little more than briefly flash a light in the mouth during the "Say Ahhh" oral examination. Unless pathology is prominent and readily apparent, looking at the tonsils is rarely even a part of the examination routine. Typically, the oral cavity is quickly noted to be "normal," even without a specific tonsillar examination as the physician proceeds with the rest of the physical examination. And as minimal as this oral examination is, a very large number of physicians don't even have their patients open their mouths at all before initiating a general workup and putting together a treatment plan for whatever medical condition is present.

Patients with recurrent tonsillitis often have discernible surface pathology on the tonsils. However, very many normal-appearing tonsils (as Issels noted above) are severely infected. While it might not identify all such infected tonsils, the application of firm pressure laterally against the tonsil and the tissue anterior to it can result in the expression of cellular debris, caseous material, and even frank pus. This should always be part of the routine physical examination, especially in adults with any heart disease, cancer, or other chronic degenerative disease.

Conclusion

Normal-appearing, chronically infected tonsils are arguably one of the most unrecognized focal infections. And as demonstrated in Chapter 3 and in Josef Issels' work with cancer patients, focal infections, such as infected tonsils, typically have a severe negative impact on the general health, because they can initiate as well as aggravate multiple health conditions. Such infections are especially problematic relative to other oral focal infections. Unlike X-ray examinations that can sometimes detect unsuspected dental infections during regular screening, there are really no routine screening tests that would "stumble" across the presence of chronically infected tonsils.

Generally, it is only the tonsils that have been ravaged by frequent bouts of tonsillitis that eventually receive enough attention to warrant being surgically removed. However, a growing body of evidence would indicate that many, if not the vast majority, of tonsils that are exposed to chronically infected teeth and gums for an extended period, eventually become chronically infected and abscessed themselves. Furthermore, it appears that when tonsils reach this degree of infection, they characteristically remain infected, even long after the infected teeth and gums that initially precipitated their infection have been extracted or otherwise been effectively treated.

Health practitioners should always consider the possibility of chronically infected tonsils playing a significant role in causing and aggravating any of the established chronic degenerative diseases. And they need to be high on the list of important considerations in the evaluation and eventual effective treatment of such conditions.

Infected Dental Implants

Overview

Dental implants are devices (usually titanium posts) that are surgically inserted into the jawbone where natural teeth are missing in order to support a dental prosthesis. The dental prosthesis can be a bridge, a denture, or the most common reason for placement of an implant, a single prosthetic tooth.[1] Physiologically, the goal of the procedure is osseointegration, meaning that the bone surrounding the implant solidly grows around and even a bit into the surface of the implant.[2,3]

There are a number of different surgical techniques for placing implants along with differing techniques for maintaining long-term mechanical integrity. Even though there are many published studies on dental implants, this procedural variability makes it difficult to make absolute statistical assertions as to the long-term stability of implants in general. Many studies investigate the success rates of various techniques, their rates of mechanical soundness, and the frequency of implant failure due to infection or inflammation. There are even investigations that document the degree to which "lesser" degrees of infection and inflammation might impact overall health. However, no studies could be found that looked at the correlation between the presence of implants, their long-term ability to function under varying degrees of infection and/or inflammation, and any impact they might be having on different chronic diseases or longevity in general. Furthermore, no studies were found that examined the impact of implants on important trackers of general health, such as C-reactive protein (CRP) or other laboratory indicators of chronic systemic inflammation.

Pathophysiology and Prevalence

Generally, dental implant disease falls into two categories. The first category (peri-implant mucositis) refers to a relatively superficial gum inflammation around the area of the implant's initial penetration into the gums. The second (peri-implantitis) is a deep-seated inflammation and/or infection at the embedded implant apex and around the portion of the implant surrounded by bone or gum tissue. Peri-implantitis is much more serious and is roughly analogous to chronic apical periodontitis (CAP) in a natural tooth.[4] Not surprisingly, the microbial profile of peri-implantitis is very similar to other periodontal infections.[5,6]

Just as with a chronically infected native tooth, the presence of periodontal pathogens and inflammation found in peri-implantitis is associated with a steady resorption of the bone around the implant concurrent with a functional deterioration of supporting bone integrity over time.[7] No significant studies could be found that looked at the correlation of implants with varying degrees of peri-implantitis to different systemic diseases or body-wide inflammation. However, one study did correlate increased cardiovascular disease with the presence and concentration of the periodontal pathogen *Prevotella intermedia* in the gum tissues below the implant insertion point (the peri-implant sulcus).[8,9]

> *There is no reason to believe that an infected implant should have a substantially different impact on general health than an infected tooth.*

Considering an infected implant's similarity to previously discussed periodontal infections, there is no reason to believe that an infected implant should have a substantially different impact on general health than an infected tooth.

There is lack of clear consensus on defining where "acceptable" degrees of peri-implant mucositis and peri-implantitis become "unacceptable" and represent a failed implant. However, a great deal of information has been published on the histology and pathogen profile of these two pathologies and the risk factors that contribute to them.

The ultimate goal in an implant procedure is to attach a dental prosthesis that maintains enough structural integrity to allow normal chewing function without pain. Beyond that goal there do not appear to be any studies directly investigating whether dental implants, diseased or not, inflict a negative impact on the general health. There are, however, studies that look at disorders that are commonly found in patients with implants (comorbidities).[10] However, since very few adults are completely disease-free, there is really no way to know whether a comorbidity is simply a coincidence or is actually related to the presence of dental implants. That will remain the case until specific studies are conducted to explore these issues.

The prevalence of inflammation at dental implant sites is quite high.

What we do know, however, is that the prevalence of inflammation at dental implant sites is quite high. In the Consensus Report of the Sixth European Workshop on Periodontology, it was concluded that peri-implant mucositis was present at 50% of implant sites examined, affecting 80% of the subjects. Peri-implantitis was identified at 12%

to 40% of implant sites, affecting between 28% and 56% of the subjects. This report indicated that common risk factors for peri-implant disease included poor oral hygiene, a history of peri-odontitis, diabetes, and smoking.[11-13] Significant peri-implantitis can lead to eventual mechanical failure of the implant, but there are many other factors that can also play a significant role in contributing to the ultimate failure of osseointegration.[14,15]

Peri-implant mucositis was present at 50% of implant sites examined, affecting 80% of the subjects.

Interestingly, the implant procedure immediately following extraction nearly always achieves a satisfactory mechanical stability outcome, at least in the early years post-procedure. Furthermore, implants placed immediately in freshly debrided sockets after the extraction of teeth with periapical pathology like CAP, also nearly always have satisfactory mechanical outcomes.[16] Meticulous debridement/cleaning of the socket with the complete removal of infected bone, along with pre- and post-surgical antibiotic therapy plays a significant role in assuring an adequate long-term, mechanical outcome.[17] Supportive healing modalities like the use of platelet-rich plasma along with ozone treatment of the socket at the time of extraction and intermittently thereafter are all also very important in assuring good healing in the socket and around the implant (osseointegration).

Some authors feel that the immediate implant procedure actually ***reduces*** the amount of bone resorption in the socket, resulting in an extraction site with a greater volume of bone long-term than when the socket is left alone until bone healing is complete. Furthermore, the patient is much happier to have the immediate availability of a tooth prosthesis in order to promptly resume normal chewing rather than waiting several months to even a year or longer before the dental prosthesis is in place and functioning normally.[18]

A literature review revealed that the ability of immediate implant placement versus "early" implant placement yielded comparable results in terms of mechanical stability of the prosthesis. However, it was also noted that there was little data available to be reviewed regarding long-term success as measured by peri-implant tissue health and prosthesis stability.[19] It has also been shown that the survival rate of immediately-placed implants with the prosthetic teeth being immediately attached ("loaded") to the implants was pretty much the same as when months were allowed to pass, presumably to allow greater osseointegration before loading of the prostheses.[20]

As implants are very expensive procedures, there are many people who cannot afford them, and the ones who can afford them (at least once) do not want to be looking at repeat procedures or proceeding to another pricey dental restoration after only a few years. Patients also deserve to know how chronic states of implant inflammation are impacting the general health, even if mechanical stability remains.

Health Impact of Peri-implantitis

As noted above, no significant examination has yet been made as to the impact of chronic peri-implantitis on general health. As long as an implant is mechanically stable and allows for pain-free chewing, the implant has presumably fulfilled its intended purpose. And perhaps it has. However, the studies still need to be performed.

Some degree of peri-implantitis and its predecessor, peri-implant mucositis, is quite common with dental implants.

A state of chronic inflammation and/or infection is never desirable anywhere in the body. However, whether a low-grade inflamed/infected implant impacts general health in the same manner as an inflamed/infected native tooth remains to be determined. It is likely that it does not, for the reason discussed immediately below. That said, it is important that such studies be performed, since some degree of peri-implantitis and its predecessor, peri-implant mucositis, is quite common with dental implants.[21-24]

Physiologically, an implant differs from a native tooth in at least one very important aspect. Unlike a native tooth, a properly-placed implant, especially after good osseointegration has occurred, does not have a facilitated access to the lymphatic and venous drainage systems in the jawbone. Generally, infected native teeth can quickly and easily express their pathogen and toxin contents into these drainage systems, and then dissemination throughout the body is free to ensue. An infected implant, however, is much more like a cavitation than a typical CAP tooth since the infection/ inflammation and its byproducts can stay in place as long as the infection has not resorbed too much bone and eaten its way too deeply into the socket area.

It is also important to realize that infected implants do not generally stay stable indefinitely.

It is also important to realize that infected implants do not generally stay stable indefinitely. Even though an infected implant may facilitate good chewing for a number of years, at some point it can reach a state of instability and advanced infection with the radiological appearance of an advanced CAP tooth. It is very important, then, that even the most mechanically sound of implants gets regular, long-term follow-up with high resolution imaging to promptly detect any new or evolving inflammation and infection. A long period of prolonged implant infection should not be allowed to elapse before being properly addressed.

The scientific literature has three follow-up designations for implants: a ***success***, a prosthesis that has ***survived***, or a ***failure***. Successful implants have no pain or tenderness, no mobility, no history of exudates, and have less than 2 mm of bone loss on X-ray since the initial placement. Surviving implants have no pain or minimal sensitivity and no mobility, but have bone losses of 2 mm to greater than 4 mm as well as the ability to probe greater than 7 mm alongside the prosthesis. A failed implant has pain and mobility, a significant exudate, and bone loss that is greater than one half the length of the implant.[25]

Despite the wide variance in implant protocols, techniques, materials, and risk factor profiles, the dental implant is statistically a very effective mechanical dental intervention. Regardless, implants usually endure for a substantial number of years. In a study that looked at 23 patients given implants 15 years earlier, researchers reported a 95% implant survival rate.[26] The same implant survival numbers were seen in a retrospective analysis of 10,000 implants followed up to

The scientific literature has three follow-up designations for implants: a success, a prosthesis that has survived, or a failure.

20 years, using implant approaches both with and without bone augmentation.[27]

Even in patients with moderate periodontitis, the survival rate of the implants placed was about 94%. Many other studies also put the implant survival rate, depending on how the study was constructed and how long the study groups were followed, between 94 and 100%. Repeat implants at sites of previously failed implants had survival rates roughly ranging from 71% to 95%. Third attempt implants had a survival rate of 74%.

The statistics on implants cited above also pertain to implants placed immediately after the extraction of teeth **with CAP!**[28-37] One of the studies even showed an excellent outcome for immediately-placed implants in extraction sites where the infection-generated granulation tissue was allowed to **remain** versus in extraction sites where it was removed. Certainly, this relatively recent data reported in the literature would indicate

Extraction followed by immediate implant placement is emerging as an effective and viable approach as well.

that in addition to the options of root canal treatment or just tooth extraction when a CAP tooth is encountered, extraction followed by immediate implant placement is emerging as an effective and viable approach as well.

While there should be no problem appreciating how a grossly infected implant with a large surrounding radiolucent area from bone resorption and infection would negatively impact the general health of the patient, it also becomes apparent that implant failure is not an overnight phenomenom. Rather, the peri-implantitis of a given implant is generally a non-linear, accelerating process, and it typically begins within the first three years.[38]

Serial CRP values should be an integral part of the routine follow-up of dental implant status.

No studies could be found that examined any correlation between increasing CRP values and increasing degrees of implant failure. Even so, it is inconceivable that the implants with the most advanced failure and most pronounced infection would not trigger significantly elevated CRP values the vast majority of the time. Certainly, an elevated CRP level is a basic screening test for orthopedic prosthetic infections.[39] It should be no different for a bone prosthesis infection in the mouth. Tooth infections of any kind generally have higher CRP levels with the more severe infections.[40] With this in mind, serial CRP values should be an integral part of the routine follow-up of dental implant status. If CRP levels continue to increase over time, and there appears to be a correlation to a worsening clinical and/or X-ray status of an implant, then vigorous intervention measures need to be applied to see if the peri-implantitis can be curbed or even be significantly reversed.

Detecting the presence and/or worsening of peri-implantitis at its earliest stages via careful 3D cone beam imaging, along with serial CRP measurements should be a part of regular follow-up care.

Such interventions of proven efficacy for varying degrees of implant failure include ozone therapy, laser decontamination, implantoplasty surgery, guided bone regeneration, and antibiotic therapy.[41-45] Once remediation has been performed, a decline in CRP level would provide substantial confidence that the implantitis-associated toxicity has been reasonably contained and that general health status is not being negatively impacted to a great degree. Detecting the presence and/or worsening of peri-implantitis at its earliest stages via careful 3D cone beam imaging, along with serial CRP measurements should be a part of regular follow-up care. These diagnostics, in conjunction with proven interventions as indicated, should reliably result in a significant improvement in the total implant survival time.[46]

Conclusion

Dental implant placement is an increasingly popular restoration technique for missing teeth. And while implants are considerably more expensive than root canal procedures, the long-term economics of an implant may actually be far less. The chronic toxicity and related health impacts of a root canal have already been demonstrated. If such a procedure is never performed, and the tooth is extracted, it can never develop CAP with the potential damage to the immune system and the provocation of any variety of diseases. Although an implant can become infected, remediation is easier and cheaper than a repeated root canal procedure, and infected implants appear to carry much less risk of seeding and feeding disease than a CAP tooth.

For the patient who insists on having a root canal treatment rather than an extraction in order not to lose chewing function, having the possibility of immediately following the extraction with a dental implant can give the patient an important additional option. The only two options need not be just tolerating a chronic infection inherent in a root canal-treated tooth in order to maintain full chewing ability versus having a toothless socket without chewing ability.

The placement of a successful dental implant has never been documented to exert any significant systemic toxicity, in contrast to the well-documented body-wide toxic impact of many root canal-treated teeth. And, it seems unlikely that well-designed studies will ever prove this to be the case. Such studies need to incorporate regular 3D cone beam imaging of the dental prostheses, along with regular CRP testing in order to best identify when implants need to be treated, or even removed when peri-implantitis and infection has made saving the implant untenable.

Finally, follow-up evaluations of placed implants are needed in order to detect and address the earliest stages of peri-implantitis prior to eventual failure and before significant systemic toxicity has had an extended period of time to damage the general health.

Cavitational Osteonecrosis

Overview

Cavitational osteonecrosis, or cavitations, are residual infected holes in the jawbone due to incomplete healing after tooth loss or extraction. While still little recognized or even appreciated as existing by mainstream dentistry, it is nevertheless an extremely prevalent condition. Having some degree of cavitation present after an extraction of one of the larger teeth is far and away the rule rather than the exception. The prevalence of cavitations after the "routine" extraction/removal of the wisdom teeth (third molars) has been studied. In a review of 112 randomly selected patients who had such old and presumably completely healed extraction sites explored directly by drill bit, cavitations were clearly present at least 88% of the time (313 of 354 sites explored). Furthermore, these explorations took place regardless of X-ray appearance, as a majority of cavitations are not apparent on screening X-ray examinations.

As some cavitations are smaller and eccentric in location, it is highly probable that the cavitation prevalence was even higher than what was found by the blind drilling approach. Generally speaking, the smaller the tooth extracted, the less the chance of finding a significant cavitation on exploration. Nevertheless, in the data that was reviewed, the overall prevalence of cavitations reported was 77% (536 out of 691 explored sites), regardless of the locations of the extracted teeth.[1]

While there remains little awareness of the substantial presence of cavitations after routine extractions, there is a small but increasing awareness of cavitation-like osteonecrosis formation as a side effect of bisphosphonate drugs. These drugs are used in the treatment of osteopenia and osteoporosis. Osteonecrosis is found to be present a small percentage of the time in bisphosphonate-treated patients who undergo subsequent dental surgery. Most commonly it occurs in cancer patients treated with this drug group, although it is also seen in treated osteoporosis patients without cancer.[2] Nevertheless, since the diagnosis and treatment of bisphosphonate-related osteonecrosis is

> *In the data that was reviewed, the overall prevalence of cavitations reported was 77%...*

largely relegated to dental specialists, the overall awareness of this dental pathology among dentists in general is still very minimal.[3]

Even though bisphosphonate-related lesions are similar to the necrosis found in post-extraction cavitations, the public health impact of the post-extraction lesions far exceeds that of post-bisphosphonate lesions. Although the treatment protocols are very similar, the reasons for the variations in clinical impact is three-fold:

The overall awareness of this dental pathology among dentists in general is still very minimal.

1. **Frequency of occurrence**. The number of individuals with post-extraction cavitations far exceeds the number with bisphosphonate-related osteonecrosis.

2. **Presence of Pathogens**. Post-extraction cavitations often occur after the extraction of an infected tooth and are exposed to an ever-present host of oral pathogens during the healing process. Bisphosphonate-related osteonecrosis evolves without any direct exposure to the pathogens of the oral cavity.

3. **Location of the pathology**. Both forms of osteonecrosis have a wide variety in size, and their proximity of the largest

lesions to the vascular and lymphatic delivery systems deep in the jawbone is very important in determining how effectively pathogens and toxins eventually disseminate throughout the body.

Unfortunately, the increased awareness of post-bisphosphonate lesions has not significantly increased awareness of post-extraction lesions (cavitations), and the need to refine the extraction procedure of teeth in order to minimize the occurrence and/or size of such lesions is still not part of standard dental protocols.

Pathophysiology

The pathological nature of cavitations was actually described long ago.[4] A typical lesion is a hollowed-out area secondary to necrosis (death) of bone structure at an old extraction site. These holes contain the non-viable debris that results from the dissolution of the bony matrix. Varying degrees of new bone breakdown can be present at any given point in time depending upon whether the defect is confined to the extraction space or extends beyond it. Some cavitations are very static, while others

> *A typical lesion is a hollowed-out area secondary to necrosis (death) of bone structure at an old extraction site.*

undergo active spread and produce larger defects over time.

Generally, cavitations have a chronic but relatively sparse microbe population that includes pathogens and their associated toxins. Since any given cavitation begins and develops amidst a unique microbial flora, no two are completely alike. This fact becomes readily apparent upon exploration and debridement.

Histologically, the contents of cavitations are very close in nature to wet gangrene.

Cavitational contents have been noted to be green, yellow-green, and even dark and tar-like. Additional reported characterizations of the contents include blood-soaked sawdust, chocolate ice cream, spongy bone, gritty powdered dust, and even green fatty globules. The consistencies are also quite variable, as they can be loose and runny in nature, or even clumped, somewhat akin to cottage cheese. Some are serous-like in nature and actually appear clear. Not surprisingly, the contents sometimes have very foul, putrid odors. Histologically, the contents of cavitations are very close in nature to wet gangrene.

The vast majority of the time a cavitation is pain-free and not even sensitive to direct pressure during an oral examination. Although it contains pathogens, toxins, and necrotic material, there is generally no increase in body temperature, and there is virtually never any associated erythema or swelling. Some upper jawbone cavitations, however, can be detected by some discomfort upon direct finger pressure to the suspected site. This local discomfort is more difficult to elicit in the lower jawbone, which has a higher bone density than the upper jawbone.

Typically, cavitations do not exhibit prominent bacterial proliferation or large numbers of inflammatory cells such as monocytes and lymphocytes. Neutrophils, which are the primary cells in abscesses and other pus-filled lesions, are conspicuously absent.

Larger cavitations that interconnect contain relatively large volumes of toxic debris, reach the draining lymphatics of the jawbone, and course over the main jawbone nerves.

Small, well-contained cavitations that have not spread to adjacent teeth or extended to the main nerve in the jawbone generally appear to have no significant systemic health impact. However, larger cavitations that interconnect contain relatively large volumes of toxic debris, reach the draining lymphatics of the jawbone, and course over the main jawbone nerves. These can produce a substantial, negative body-wide impact on general health.

Studies have yet to be done that correlate cavitations to elevations of CRP (C-reactive protein), which reflect increases in systemic inflammation and increased oxidative stress throughout the body. Perhaps smaller cavitations have no impact on CRP and only affect this test when they exceed a certain size, or perhaps the CRP has a graded and linear increase that relates directly to cavitation size. This remains to be determined, but such a study will be of great value in evaluating whether smaller cavitations can be safely ignored, or whether they still warrant surgical debridement and revision.

...a neuralgia-inducing cavitational osteonecrosis (NICO) lesion...can cause a significant negative impact on general health.

There is, however, a rare but highly symptomatic type of cavitation called a neuralgia-inducing cavitational osteonecrosis (NICO) lesion that can cause a significant negative impact on general health.[5] A NICO is a large cavitation that reaches the main nerve in the jawbone and generally involves a much larger quantity of necrotic, toxic material than the typical cavitation. The associated pain is often severe and often radiates backward toward the trigeminal nerve. Much of the time inflammation and damage to the sheath surrounding the affected nerves (demyelination) can take place and antimyelin antibodies can be present. Demyelination is not always a result, however, since other mechanisms, such as increased pressure in the affected areas containing the nerves, can cause inflammation and pain without initiating frank nerve damage.[6]

Most likely NICO lesions are accompanied by CRP elevations much or most of the time, although no study was found that investigated this inflammation biomarker in patients with NICO. There is, however, evidence that NICO lesions do have systemic inflammatory impact as a host of defects of the thrombotic and fibrinolytic systems,

Samples from such cavitation lesions show high levels of inflammatory messengers, and these messengers have been found in high titer in some patients with breast cancer and advanced neurological illnesses.

along with some defective immune responses, have been identified in many NICO patients.[7] It would appear that not only do extensive cavitations negatively impact the clotting mechanisms of the body, but defects in these mechanisms also promote the formation of cavitations. Furthermore, there is evidence that surgical debridement of cavitations can lead to improvement in a number of conditions associated with chronic inflammation. Samples from such cavitation lesions show high levels of inflammatory messengers, and these messengers have been found in high titer in some patients with breast cancer and advanced neurological illnesses.[8]

Perhaps the primary reason that cavitations are so common is because the "standard" technique of tooth extraction greatly facilitates cavitation development. Most extractions take place because a tooth becomes infected and remains painful. Very few extractions take place outside of the context of an ongoing infection, except when teeth are removed for orthodontic reasons, to facilitate the fitting of full dentures, or to prevent problems with wisdom teeth. Even in the case of an older person who is receiving dentures, it is still more common than not that the few remaining teeth to be extracted are still associated with some degree of periodontitis and local infection. However, uninfected wisdom teeth extractions also have very high prevalence of cavitations.

In addition to infection often being present in the tooth socket at the time of extraction, the typical extraction makes no attempt to remove the periodontal ligament that surrounds the tooth in the bony socket. The periodontal ligament is a thin yet dense connective tissue that lines the socket, helps to anchor the tooth to the surrounding bone, and serves to act as a shock absorber to minimize the force and trauma of chewing. When this ligament is not specifically targeted for removal as part of the extraction procedure, part, or all, of the ligament typically remains after the tooth is removed.

However, after the tooth has been removed and the ligament remains, the surrounding bone abutting the ligament has no physiological "awareness" that the tooth is gone. This bone does not naturally grow through the ligament to fill the socket site with new bone, and the ligament does not generally spontaneously resorb. However, sometimes part of the ligament remains attached to the tooth and that part of it tears away and is inadvertently removed as a part of the extraction process. When this occurs, some bone usually grows in where the ligament was removed, but complete socket healing still does not occur. This helps to account for why cavitations have such a variety of sizes and shapes, since any two extractions rarely occur in a technically identical manner.

What does happen most of the time, then, is that the top of the extraction site has no periodontal ligament, and the bone gradually re-grows a thin cap of bone that covers the defect. As mentioned previously, many extractions start with teeth that are already infected and result in infected bone deep in the socket. At the time of extraction, the microbial flora of the mouth also has an extended period of time to get a foothold inside the socket before the thin cap of bone has an opportunity to completely grow over and seal off the extraction site defect. When healing of the cap of bone atop the extraction site is complete, the enclosed defect is officially a cavitation without any mechanism to restore a sterile state. Instead, multiple microbes have been contained, many of them aerobic bacteria in a new anaerobic environment.

Such anaerobic trapping makes many benign bacteria become highly pathogenic via the secretion of potent exotoxins. The bacterial pathophysiology involved is much the same as what happens when an organism like *Clostridium botulinum* gets trapped in the anaerobic environment of a vacuum-packed can of food. At that point, the bacteria begin to form the highly potent botulinum toxin. Virtually harmless to man in the presence of oxygen, such a species of bacteria can quickly become deadly when the oxygen is removed and the toxin is formed. So, even when extraction sites do not start infected, which is nevertheless usually the case, they can be expected to become infected.

Any properly performed extraction must involve a deliberate debridement of the socket until healthy bone is reached, after which a normal blood clot can form and begin the process of normal healing. Along with the proper cleaning of the socket, the use of a post-extraction therapy like platelet-rich plasma strongly supports good healing.[9-12] Ozone treatments support good healing as well.

An additional factor that promotes cavitation formation following tooth extraction is the use of local anesthetics with vasoconstrictor agents such as epinephrine. Vasoconstriction narrows the blood vessels and slows the blood flow in the injected area, which results in a longer period of time being needed to wash out the anesthetic agent. This effect also makes it easier to control bleeding, generally a desirable effect for most surgical procedures. However, this vasoconstriction can result in inadequate blood supply (ischemia) around the borders of the extraction site which promotes the death of more bone than is necessary and makes the resulting extraction defect larger. Relative to the soft tissues, bone is even more sensitive to the negative impact of the ischemia that can be induced by vasoconstrictor agents.

Many edentulous individuals, when surgically explored in the course of debridement, have an extensive cavitation burden.

Unfortunately, the vast majority of dental extractions are done without any regard to the above considerations, and the wet gangrene-containing holes in the jawbone known as cavitations routinely result. Not surprisingly, the toxicity of cavitations depends on the total cavitation burden that is present. For example an edentulous (no teeth) person would have a greater cavitation burden than an individual who had one extracted tooth. Many edentulous individuals, when surgically explored in the course of debridement, have an extensive cavitation burden. Often there is much interconnection between and among the old extraction sites, often appearing in a channel-like fashion throughout the jawbone rather than as an interrupted sequence of focal cavitation sites. Also, the degree to which single cavitations have spread and acquired the characteristics of NICO lesions, as discussed above, is also very important in determining the systemic health impact of cavitations.

Health Impact of Cavitations

Since cavitations remain an entity that is unknown to the vast majority of dentists and physicians, it should not be surprising that there are no studies that directly examine the associations between cavitations and different chronic diseases. Nevertheless, there does exist data that clearly demonstrates a profoundly negative impact of the larger cavitations, as with NICO, and a greater collective cavitation burden on longevity in general and cardiac health in particular.

In this context, multiple studies have been performed that inadvertently make the case for the significant toxicity of cavitations and the negative impact they can have on the body. Although none of the authors cited indicate any awareness of the prevalence and systemic toxicity of cavitations, it has been established that toothless individuals have a significantly increased all-cause mortality compared to individuals who still have teeth.[13] Furthermore, the effect is graded such that persons with less teeth have an increased all-cause mortality than persons with more teeth, but not necessarily a full set of teeth.[14-18] Another study found increased all-cause mortality correlated not only with less teeth but also with more periodontal disease in the remaining teeth, a logical outcome when considering cumulative toxic burden.[19] While tooth replacement or dentures would be expected to provide improved nutrition, it does not yet appear to have been demonstrated that it can negate or significantly mitigate the toxic impact of the cavitation burden present.[20]

While cavitations do not generally have as much active inflammation and infection as many other dental and oral cavity infections, the pathogen and toxin profiles are pretty much the same. Just as there is a cause-and-effect relationship between heart attacks and the oral pathogens of root canal-treated teeth and infected gums, the statistical data would also indicate a strong relationship between heart attacks and patients with a high cavitation burden. And while high cavitation burdens clearly correlate with increased all-cause mortality, it would appear there is even a stronger correlation with death from coronary artery disease.[21-24]

None of the studies cited even considered the fact that in the course of losing teeth or eventually becoming edentulous there also had to be a substantial loss of chronically infected teeth in the form of root canal-treated teeth or asymptomatic CAP teeth. This reality dramatically further highlights the impact of cavitation toxicity on cardiac and all-cause mortality. As demonstrated earlier, such teeth can have an enormously negative impact on health and longevity, and it has also been shown that most adults have at least a few such infected teeth. Yet, even when such teeth have been removed, it would appear that a large amount of residual cavitation toxicity still has more negative clinical impact than would have been realized by leaving a few infected teeth unextracted. However, when proper extraction techniques finally become commonplace and collective cavitation burdens are minimized, it should result in edentulous individuals having a lowered all-cause mortality.

Conclusion

Cavitational osteonecrosis is an extremely common dental condition, and nearly 90% of the extraction sites of wisdom teeth end up with significant cavitations. This means that effectively everyone who has had all four wisdom teeth extracted has at least one cavitation, but much more likely between two and four. Even though cavitations remain little recognized by mainstream dentistry, they nevertheless represent a significant public health problem by themselves, especially when they are large, multiple, or extending throughout the jawbone, as is seen in many edentulous patients. A great deal of data leads to the conclusion that a greater cavitation burden results in a significantly increased all-cause mortality.

It also appears that mortality from coronary heart disease is even more strongly impacted by increased cavitation burden than many other chronic degenerative diseases. It is important, then, that the diagnosis of cavitations is vigorously pursued, and surgical debridement of these old extraction sites should be a much more common procedure than is currently the case. This would especially be true when CRP levels remain persistently elevated after other oral cavity infections and/or focal infections throughout the body have been effectively diagnosed and addressed. Intermittent ozone injections into cavitations in conjunction with, or even preceding, surgical debridement can be very valuable in making residual defects smaller, even if they do not get completely eradicated. For some individuals with smaller cavitations, intermittent ozone injection is proving to be a potential stand-alone therapy.

Infected Sinuses

Overview

There are three paranasal, bony sinuses with a minimal potential for serious health impact: the frontal located just above the eyebrows, the ethmoidal behind the bridge of the nose, and the sphenoidal directly behind the ethmoidal sinus. However, because of their proximity to the upper jawbones (maxillae), the maxillary sinuses are the most significant as sites of focal infections. As such, when these sinuses are infected, they can have a serious negative impact on health.

Maxillary sinuses are the bony air-filled cavities located under the cheekbones and directly above the maxillae. They are of primary importance because they are far more likely to become chronically inflamed and infected from an adjacent infected tooth, a periodontal infection, or a cavitation than the other sinuses.

Unfortunately, the frequent association between maxillary sinus infection and these dental pathologies remains rarely suspected. Even though such a connection could be easily identified with 3D cone beam imaging of the sinuses and the maxillary teeth sockets, patients with chronic sinus infections are not routinely examined for a potential dental infection. Consequently, many individuals receive symptom-treating medical and even surgical therapies that never fully remediate the sinus infection because the underlying dental pathology is never evaluated and addressed.

Unfortunately, the frequent association between maxillary sinus infection and these dental pathologies remains rarely suspected.

It is just as important that the ENT (ear, nose, and throat) medical specialist obtain 3D cone beam dental examination of the patient as it is for the dentist. This should be routine in the initial workup, although periodic follow-up examinations are also very important since "new" teeth can become asymptomatically infected at any point in time.

Pathophysiology

Maxillary sinus disease often occurs as part of a broader clinical syndrome known as chronic rhinosinusitis, a syndrome characterized by continued inflammation of the nose and paranasal sinuses. In the scientific literature it is still acknowledged as a condition that is poorly understood pathophysiologically.[1] Multiple factors have been researched as being significant players in causing this condition, including persistent bacterial biofilms, autoimmune diseases, allergens, toxins, and defects in the host immune system.[2-5] Symptoms can range widely from occasional runny nose and sneezing to intermittent or even chronic infections in the sinuses, with facial pain and pus accumulation. Once maxillary disease is advanced, most patients turn to an internist and/or ENT specialist for further diagnosis and treatment.

Until ruled out, it should always be suspected that an infected or inflamed tooth in the upper jawbone is causing or strongly contributing to maxillary sinusitis. The CAP tooth in the maxilla is generally asymptomatic, even though the local and systemic toxicity might be great. 3D cone beam imaging of the upper jawbone teeth should

3D cone beam imaging of the upper jawbone teeth should always be obtained in the workup of acute maxillary sinusitis...

always be obtained in the workup of acute maxillary sinusitis, and it is just as important to do it in the patient who has chronic maxillary sinusitis, no matter how many specialists have been involved in the care of that patient over the years.

The very fact that the condition is chronic and has never definitively responded to a treatment protocol is additional evidence that a chronically infected tooth (or dental implant) is possibly causing the condition. A study that reviewed maxillofacial computed tomography studies in 171 maxillary sinuses diagnosed with acute maxillary sinusitis found 16% of the cases had CAP, and 71% of the cases had projecting tooth roots, meaning inflammation secondary to tooth pathology was present more than 75% of the time.[6]

...with acute maxillary sinusitis... inflammation secondary to tooth pathology was present more than 75% of the time.

In a related case report, a 41-year-old male presented with chronic sinusitis of nine years duration. His related symptoms included nasal congestion, post-nasal drip, throat clearing, headaches, and pain/pressure over the cheek area. Although a CT scan revealed an erupted molar tooth projecting into the left maxillary sinus, an ENT surgical approach to the sinus was initially done that included septoplasty (a surgical procedure to straighten a deviated septum). After an initial improvement, all symptoms returned, and a purulent discharge ensued that persisted in spite of multiple courses of antibiotics. Sixteen months later, repeat CT scan showed that sinus to be completely filled, and a first molar cyst was seen extending up into the sinus. Repeat sinus surgery that included extraction of the involved molar tooth with granuloma was then performed. Following a repeat course of antibiotics, the infection resolved along with all associated inflammatory changes. The patient then had a complete recovery.[7]

Although the case report above involved only one patient, it demonstrates a pathology that is very common in patients with chronic sinusitis. Nevertheless, the evaluation of the maxillary teeth in patients with maxillary sinusitis is not routinely performed. The infected tooth-infected sinus connection appears to be no more widely appreciated than the fact that many teeth with chronic infection exist and remain undetected. Most likely this is because these infections are frequently asymptomatic and 3D cone beam dental examinations have yet to become a routine part of dental and medical workups.

The infected tooth-infected sinus connection appears to be no more widely appreciated than the fact that many teeth with chronic infection exist and remain undetected.

When an ENT surgeon discovers dental involvement during CT examination, in the course of mapping out the surgical approach to an inflamed/infected sinus, additional dental interventions are usually indicated. A much stronger connection of dental pathology to chronic sinus disease is now being realized as 3D cone beam imaging is increasingly employed.

Prior to the regular use of CT scanning and later the use of 3D cone beam imaging, chronic maxil-

lary sinusitis was felt to be secondary to dental
pathology only about 10 to 12% of the time.[8,9] As
this sophisticated imaging technology was utilized
more routinely, studies revealed that as many as
45% of chronic maxillary sinusitis cases had associated dental pathology in the upper jawbone.

Significant mucosal thickening in the sinuses
in conjunction with dental pathology was seen in
61% of the patients in one retrospective analysis
of 3D cone beam imaging scans. This indicates that
dental pathology might well be responsible for the
majority of chronic sinusitis cases.[10-14] When significant fluid opacification of the affected sinus is
present, moderate mucosal thickening was found in
one study to have associated dental pathology 86%
of the time.[15] Another study that examined unilateral sinus opacification found associated dental
pathology 73% of the time.[16]

Even when regular CT imaging reveals no
obvious dental pathology, unilateral maxillary
sinusitis should still raise a high level of concern
that there is still some underlying dental pathology
as an etiology. In such cases 3D cone beam imaging
is still advisable, along with standard testing to see
if selected maxillary teeth are viable.[17]

Health Impact of Infected Sinuses

As anywhere else in the body, a chronic inflam-
mation/infection in the sinus can be expected to
negatively impact the general health of the body.
The degree of impact will depend on a number of

factors. These include how advanced the infection might be, its access to lymphatic drainage for potential dissemination throughout the body, and the immunocompetence of the individual with the infection.

In reviewing the literature, no significant studies were found that have investigated the impact of chronic maxillary sinusitis on general health, or its impact and correlation with specific diseases. Probably the main reason for this is that acute or chronic sinusitis is an inflammation/infection with symptoms that get the attention of both the patient and the healthcare professional (physician and/or dentist), which is not the case with most focal infections. As such, it is a problem that generally can be resolved when addressed correctly, and not typically a hidden, asymptomatic infection like a painless CAP tooth. However, one study did show that asymptomatic chronic sinusitis incidentally detected on brain magnetic resonance scans appears to have an association with cerebrovascular atherosclerosis, although not atherosclerosis in general.[18]

As an inflamed/infected sinus does not have the same venous and lymphatic drainage as an infected tooth, it should be expected that the area receiving the most pathogen/toxin drainage will be disproportionately affected, which would appear to be the cerebral circulation for the maxillary sinuses. A case report consistent with this thinking showed that a complication of cerebral abscess resulted from maxillary and frontal sinusitis.[19]

Since chronic sinusitis can exist in an asymptomatic state and still have potentially significant negative clinical impact, as with the case report on sinusitis and cerebral abscess noted above, having an additional diagnostic technique for this condition is important. There now exists a low-cost, handheld technology for imaging the maxillary sinuses taken from an intraoral approach. This diagnostic tool is known as near-infrared (NIR) optical imaging with computer analysis enhancement. The sinuses can be transilluminated, effectively allowing the differentiation of normal sinus anatomy, mild sinus disease with associated mucosal thickening, and complete sinus opacification. Additionally, the examination can be performed quickly and easily and without exposing the patient to any radiation.[20]

Chronic sinusitis, especially when unilateral, often means there is an occult infected tooth in the maxillary jawbone capable of causing great damage to the general health...

As already indicated above, chronic sinusitis, especially when unilateral, often means there is an occult infected tooth in the maxillary jawbone capable of causing great damage to the general health—including increasing the chances of heart attack and cancer. As such, then, the main significance of an infected sinus is that it effectively shines a spotlight on the possibility of involvement from a CAP tooth or other dental infection. If such a tooth is identified, it must be properly addressed to offer the best chances of achieving optimal long-term health.

While a full 3D cone beam examination of the teeth is always a good idea whenever sinusitis is part of the clinical picture, it is absolutely mandated when such sinusitis becomes chronic and will not resolve completely with an appropriate treatment protocol. In a retrospective case series of 55 patients already identified with sinusitis secondary to dental pathology, 35% of the interpreted radiology reports failed to identify or mention the presence of such pathology. This means that X-ray examinations interpreted by even the most experienced and qualified individuals cannot be used as definitive reassurance that the sinuses are normal.[21] The most current scientific data arguably indicates that a doctor and/or dentist should always look for dental pathology when sinusitis is present.

While maxillary sinusitis can develop when the roots of CAP teeth are adjacent to the sinus, it can also occur after maxillary jawbone dental implants are placed. Generally, this is the case when chronic inflammation/infection is present or even when a frank eruption of the implant tip into the sinus space is present, a good possibility if there was inadequate bone present at the start of the implant procedure.[22,23] In fact, the onset of sinusitis at some point in time after dental implant placement usually required surgical treatment to resolve the sinusitis and permit implant survival.[24]

Conclusion

Asymptomatic chronic sinusitis has the potential to significantly impact general health including increased risk of heart attack and cancer. Mainly, this is because patients with this condition rarely seek medical care.

On the other hand, chronic sinusitis that drives an individual to seek care is potentially a warning sign of the presence of a CAP tooth or other dental infection. This is particularly likely if the sinus infection is unilateral. For that reason dental involvement should always be investigated in these cases. While a full 3D cone beam examination of the teeth is always a good idea whenever sinusitis is part of the clinical picture, it is absolutely mandated when such sinusitis becomes chronic and will not resolve completely with an appropriate treatment protocol.

Logically, considering the prevalence of dental pathology's link to sinus infections demonstrated above, unsatisfactory long-term results will be commonplace as long as traditional ENT medical and/or surgical procedures are the sole approaches to chronic sinusitis. Satisfactory outcomes will likely result when specific efforts are made to identify and remediate any dental infections that are discovered.

The Diagnosis and Management of Oral Infections

Overview

Although already covered throughout the book, this chapter will serve as a concise reference that suggests a systematic process for diagnosing, treating, and managing oral infections in the patient with any chronic disease. Unique factors, such as genetic predispositions, environmental considerations, age, gender, hormonal status, and lifestyle habits, mean that no two patients are completely alike. Therefore a methodical initial workup of a patient with any chronic degenerative disease is imperative. Equally important is a clear algorithm/protocol for the ongoing follow-up evaluation and treatment of that patient on a long-term basis.

A great deal of debilitating disease-related symptomatology and needless immune system damage can be avoided by looking for worsening diagnostic parameters before obvious clinical deterioration takes place. These include objective changes that can be seen by monitoring blood test values and by comparison of periodic X-ray imaging of focal infection sites as well as 3D cone beam imaging results. And while this applies to the management of all chronic diseases, it is especially important in the ongoing management of coronary heart disease and cancers of the head, neck, and chest, especially breast cancer.

*...the evidence previously presented makes a strong argument that any first time dental or medical patient evaluation should **always** include certain baseline testing.*

Initial Patient Evaluation

Clinicians will certainly differ on how extensively a new patient should be evaluated, especially when the presenting problem is a condition that is readily resolved and/or controlled. However, the evidence previously presented makes a strong argument that any first time dental or medical patient evaluation should **always** include certain baseline testing. Even completely normal results are of great importance in the evaluation and management of that same patient in the future, when significant symptoms or clear-cut diseases begin to manifest. With this in mind, baseline evaluation should include, but not necessarily be limited to:

- ✓ **3D cone beam imaging of the teeth and associated oral cavity structures.** This will help establish the presence of any significant asymptomatic pathology (CAP—chronic apical periodontitis) at the outset, and whether blood test abnormalities are reflective of a body-wide inflammation as well. Future examinations will then reveal whether such pathology, if not immediately treated, remains stable, worsens (enlarges) or lessens over time.

- ✓ **Standard panoramic X-ray imaging** would also be of use if any pathology seen on 3D exam could also be seen on this form of X-ray, as this testing could be repeated more frequently in follow-up examinations. However, if cost is not an important consideration, follow-up 3D examinations give much more information and actually result in less radiation exposure. Also, if pathology is

...if cost is not an important consideration, follow-up 3D examinations give much more information and actually result in less radiation exposure.

detected in a specific tooth, 2D digital X-ray examinations of only that tooth can be used in follow-up rather than regular 3D exams.

✓ **Baseline blood testing** should include the following:

1. CBC and biochemistry panel, which includes the testing that tracks metabolic syndrome abnormalities (glucose, cholesterol [HDL, LDL, and total], and triglycerides), the worsening of which nearly always precedes the development of coronary atherosclerosis, especially when the baseline numbers were completely normal.

2. Lipoprotein (a)

3. ANA and RF (antinuclear antibody and rheumatoid factor)

4. Thyroid panel (including free T3 and reverse T3 levels)

5. Sex hormone levels (very important, but often overlooked in younger individuals)

6. Parameters of chronic inflammation, especially C-reactive protein (CRP); cytokine and interleukin levels would also be useful, but are costly

7. Ferritin, in order to track iron content in the body
8. Vitamin D level

✓ **Computed tomography of the coronary arteries**. This produces a computer-generated coronary artery calcium (CAC) score. While not mandatory in younger patients, the CAC score very effectively tracks whether a given treatment protocol is lessening body-wide inflammation and decreasing all-cause mortality. Although it is only the coronary calcium that is being measured, this test reflects body-wide calcium deposition and systemically increased oxidative stress. A numerical calcium score that clearly lowers when re-checked six months to a year later indicates that systemic oxidative stress was definitely lessened during that period of time. An increase in the score, however, definitely means that optimal treatment has not been rendered. And even though a truly normal calcium score is zero, a significant drop in score, such as from a 500 to a 200, indicates that treatment is positively impacting the body.

✓ **Testing appropriate for tracking a specific disease**, if the patient first presents with a chronic disease, where interval change can reflect whether the disease is responding well to the overall treatment protocol. For example, many cancer patients have associated tumor marker tests. Examples of such tests include alpha-fetoprotein, CEA, CA15-3, CA19-9, PSA, CD 20, and beta-hCG. Similarly, radionuclide scanning studies can be repeated when initially abnormal.

...optimal management requires diligence on the part of the clinician, and periodic re-evaluations should be performed even when the patient reports having no problems.

This initial evaluation may clearly indicate a medical condition that should be addressed. But, even if it is normal, it is of great value because a normal evaluation provides an important baseline for detecting and monitoring future abnormalities. Periodic repeat blood testing can readily reveal the early and subtle beginnings of a disease or medical problem—declines which are rarely detected by even the most careful annual physical examination. An abnormal blood test should trigger further evaluation, such as repeat 3D cone beam imaging of the oral cavity.

Once the manifestation of a chronic disease has been detected, optimal management requires diligence on the part of the clinician, and periodic re-evaluations should be performed even when the patient reports having no problems. Obviously, this is of particular importance in the older patient, who will likely develop one or more life-threatening problems in the future. The clinician should always aim to minimize further suffering while reasonably extending life by being proactive in patient follow-up.

As discussed earlier, significant oral cavity infections come in the form of the following:

1. Teeth that have never received a root canal procedure, with CAP
2. Root canal-treated teeth with CAP
3. Root canal-treated teeth without CAP
4. Chronic periodontal (gum and tooth-supportive tissue) disease
5. Infected tonsils
6. Infected dental implants
7. Cavitational osteonecrosis
8. Infected sinuses

Statistically, the first four types of infection are the predominant sources of oral cavity focal infections that increase general inflammation throughout the body and ultimately and quite substantially compromise general health. By itself, chronic periodontitis is a serious oral focal infection, and it is often a precursor to frank infection in the teeth. Based on the CAP prevalence studies cited in

Chapter 1, chronic periodontitis is likely often accompanied by asymptomatic infected teeth, further contributing to the strong connection between this condition and so many chronic diseases. When the appropriate studies are eventually done, there is an excellent possibility that chronic periodontitis will be shown to have a **_cause-and-effect_** relationship, not just an association, to most of those diseases for which it has already been shown to be consistently related.

Although chronically infected tonsils can significantly contribute to ill health, addressing the infected teeth should take priority.

Although chronically infected tonsils can significantly contribute to ill health, addressing the infected teeth should take priority. If after resolving dental infections, significant positive clinical and laboratory responses are not seen, then attention should refocus on the tonsils. From Dr. Issels' work, it would appear that tonsils exposed to root canal-treated teeth and CAP teeth in general leaves them chronically infected, even long after the dental pathology has been properly treated.

However, the clinician should not automatically assume that tonsillar infection is disseminating and causing body-wide inflammation unless the remediation of dental infections fails to produce a substantial improvement in the indicators of body-wide inflammation. If the CRP remains elevated, blood tests do not improve, and the clinical picture remains largely unchanged, then the tonsils must be addressed.

Treating Tooth Infections

Any teeth with clear X-ray evidence of significant infection at the root tips (chronic apical periodontitis, or CAP) should be treated, including teeth that have received root canal procedures. This is especially true when such teeth are present in the patient with a significantly elevated CRP (>3.0) and a clinical picture indicating an unstable or evolving chronic disease, such as is seen in the later stages of heart disease or cancer. The appropriate treatment can incorporate any of the following approaches, following the guidelines in Appendix B when extraction and/or the cleaning of associated cavitations is indicated:

✓ **Tooth extraction**
✓ **Tooth extraction immediately followed by a dental implant**. When technically successful, this is probably the optimal approach. Since this option is unquestionably the most expensive, the individual circumstances may render a root canal treatment the most viable option. Even if a root canal treatment is initially performed as a treatment,

should it begin to fail, extraction followed by implant still remains an option.

✓ **Root canal treatment** (not recommended as the first intervention of choice, but can be of significant benefit when patient refuses extraction and/or cannot afford an implant procedure). However, it is very important that the root canal procedure be performed by a skilled endodontist to thoroughly clean and fill the entire root canal system, not a general dentist who performs a far smaller number of these procedures. A poorly-performed root canal does not alleviate the infectious/toxic burden on the body, whereas a well-done root canal may eliminate the ability of that focus of infection to cause body-wide damage.

✓ **Recurrent ozone treatments** in and around the root tips, usually done in conjunction with a new root canal treatment, or in an effort to "stabilize" an earlier procedure before proceeding directly to extraction. If repeated ozone treatment can substantially improve pertinent blood tests, especially CRP levels, there can be an additional option of closely monitoring that tooth. This approach can also be used for the

CAP tooth that has never been given a root canal procedure, if the volume of infection is small and the blood tests look good, for the patient who simply cannot afford a dental procedure. However, it is still best for the health of the patient to extract such a tooth or give it a quality root canal procedure. Furthermore, when follow-up is careful and ongoing, such a tooth might be left alone for an indeterminate period and later extracted or given a root canal if the X-ray picture worsens along with the worsening of blood tests.

If repeated ozone treatment can substantially improve pertinent blood tests...there can be an additional option of closely monitoring that tooth.

- ✓ **Recurrent ozone injections** directly into the tonsils
- ✓ **Concurrent applications** of any of a number of protocols for lessening/resolving chronic periodontitis

As mentioned in previous chapters, an optimally-performed root canal procedure can debulk the infection that has accumulated at the root tips, while preventing ongoing leakage of any remaining pathogens and toxins if a good seal of the root canal space was achieved. However, it is impossible to determine the long-term impact of the procedure in advance. Such a root canal procedure may resolve the initial negative clinical impact and remain relatively inert for the remainder of the patient's lifetime. Or, it might become very hazardous to immediate and/or long-term health by ramping up inflammation and oxidative stress throughout the body. A possible practical approach to determining how much of a negative impact a root canal-treated tooth will have on the general health, and especially on heart disease and breast cancer, would be as follows:

✓ Evolution of blood testing results
✓ Evolution of X-ray imaging (3D or 2D digital subtraction examination of the specific tooth)
✓ Clinical evolution of chronic diseases

Ultimately, however, research studies need to be performed to see how reliably an approach like the one being suggested can reliably differentiate between root canal-treated tooth that are clinically benign and those that cause or strongly contribute to the evolution of chronic degenerative diseases like heart disease and cancer.

Evolution of Blood Testing Results

A "successful" root canal procedure should always be attended by blood testing that shows improvement, or at the very least, no worsening. In particular, this refers to the blood examinations associated with metabolic syndrome, noted above, along with the CRP level. Once the acute inflammation of healing following the procedure has subsided, usually by about one month or so, these blood values should NEVER be clearly worsened. If they have worsened, prompt extraction should be seriously considered. If prompt extraction is not deemed appropriate, for whatever reason, aggressive ozone treatments in and around the tooth apex might be performed. If, however, weekly ozone treatments for a month or so do not at least bring the blood testing results back to where they were at the time of the procedure, delaying extraction for longer periods of time needlessly exposes the patient to the destabilization of underlying diseases, including the worsening of atherosclerosis and/or the onset and/or evolution of breast cancer and other diseases.

A "successful" root canal procedure should always be attended by blood testing that shows improvement, or at the very least, no worsening.

Furthermore, a "repeat" root canal procedure should never be performed, unless the first treatment was poorly performed due to lack of expertise, and the root system was not completely cleaned and sealed. All repeat procedures should be performed

by a skilled endodontist. However, if the first procedure was performed by a skilled endodontist, a repeat procedure is never really advisable. Generally,
anatomic variability in root configurations make
the sealing of some root canal
spaces difficult to impossible
to achieve, and repeat procedures needlessly expose
the patient to pathogens and
potent toxins for months to
years longer.

*...the **interval change** in CRP levels after an intervention such as a root canal procedure is of paramount concern.*

With regard to the CRP
test, the reference range is 0
to 3.0. For the most part, this
test rises linearly in response
to greater degrees of inflam-
mation throughout the body (1.0 is worse than 0.5,
2.0 is worse than 1.5, etc.). While levels less than
0.5 are optimal, levels of 3.0 or more should always
raise concern, especially with regard to the eventual development of heart disease or cancer. And, as
alluded to above, the ***interval change*** in CRP levels
after an intervention such as a root canal procedure
is of paramount concern. A CRP that goes from 1.0
to 3.0 is likely of more concern than a CRP that goes
from 2.8 to 3.2, even though the last level is a little
higher. However, the clinician should never be comfortable accepting any CRP that chronically remains
above 3.

Evolution of X-ray Imaging

Radiolucencies around the root tips of root canal-treated teeth always indicate the presence of infections. Previously cited studies show that these "dark" areas on X-ray are clearly and reliably revealed by 3D cone beam imaging of the oral cavity, and the data in these studies suggests that at least 75% and more likely 90 to 95% of root canal-treated teeth have some degree of CAP. However, many of these studies would indicate that smaller degrees of CAP, especially if they are stable and not increasing in size over time (and even better when decreasing in size over time) may be clinically inconsequential. This is especially likely when CRP is low, blood test results are stable or improving, and both sex and thyroid hormone levels are maintained in the normal range.

Depending on multiple factors, *__some__* individuals can "wall-off" infections, including symptom-free infected teeth, and have little to no dissemination of their contents, such as might be seen with some root canals that have only small degrees of CAP. Many such teeth with CAP, however, do not have this ability and are unable to prevent pathogen/toxin dissemination, resulting in the development and evolution of many chronic diseases. It is to be expected that this is much more likely to be the case when the CAP remains large, or even grows in size after the root canal procedure, but this has not been established in any controlled studies.

Therefore, regular follow-up laboratory testing and clinical evaluation, along with properly performed and interpreted 3D cone beam imaging and/or 2D digital X-rays of specific teeth _must_ _be_ performed indefinitely to best safeguard the health of the patient.

It is important to remember that current dental and medical literature demonstrates that root canal-related pathogens directly cause most heart attacks, and that having one or more root canal-treated teeth in the mouth statistically increases the chances of having a heart attack. Consequently, even if the parameters noted above remain stable or even improve after the procedure, recommending root canal treatment as the only reasonable option can be legally problematic for the dentist in the absence of a fully informed consent. It is essential that the current literature be reviewed with the patient, and that the patient alone makes the final decision whether to proceed with the procedure.

Clinical Evolution of Chronic Diseases

It is unlikely that a given chronic disease will clearly worsen while laboratory testing and diagnostic imaging are clearly improving. Nevertheless, much remains to be learned on the optimal management of patients with chronic disease, and a clear clinical downturn should never be ignored, even if blood tests and X-rays look great. Some patients might have genetic predispositions that facilitate the development of disease with much lower pathogen titer and toxin quantities. All of these factors and considerations absolutely mandate that dentists and physicians interact much more frequently and meaningfully on behalf of their patients than is currently the standard of practice.

Treating Other Oral Cavity Infections

When infected teeth have been properly addressed and the overall health status of the patient has not clearly improved, any other oral cavity infections must be identified and treated. As periodontal disease and infected/inflamed implants are easily identified and usually very responsive to an appropriate treatment protocol, this refers to infected tonsils and sinuses, as well as to the infection in jawbone cavitations. Since various ways to diagnose and treat these infections have been presented previously, what follows are simply some additional treatment considerations.

Sinuses

Covered in some detail in Chapter 10, acute and chronic sinus infections often are due to infected teeth in the upper jawbone. Once it has been determined that all such infected teeth have been properly addressed, it is appropriate to refer the patient to the ENT (ear, nose, and throat) specialist. What is not a good idea, however, is to have extensive ENT treatments, including surgery, for any chronic sinusitis that has not first been evaluated with 3D cone beam imaging of the upper jawbone. It should be part of routine ENT evaluation to refer the patient for a screening 3D X-ray examination to look for associated/causative dental pathology and infections before any further workup or treatment is contemplated.

> *It should be part of routine ENT evaluation to refer the patient for a screening 3D X-ray examination to look for associated/causative dental pathology and infections before any further workup or treatment is contemplated.*

Cavitations

Covered in detail in Chapter 9, cavitations can range anywhere from being clinically inconsequential to being clinically overwhelmingly consequential. As such, it is a condition that should never be overlooked after the other oral cavity infections have been appropriately addressed. Much less data is available to guide cavitation diagnosis and treatment compared to the other oral cavity infections. It is likely that the same laboratory and clinical parameters will apply to significant cavitation disease as to the other oral cavity infections. When identified and there is evidence of widespread increased inflammation throughout the body, as with an elevated CRP, cavitations should be treated with ozone injections and usually surgery as well.

Tonsils

The same parameters of laboratory testing and clinical status apply to tonsillar infections as to infected teeth, as discussed above. When these parameters remain substantially abnormal, and any infected teeth and other oral cavity infections have been addressed (including sinuses and cavitations), then the tonsils need to be specifically addressed. A series of direct ozone injections should always be a part of the initial approach, and if the CRP and other laboratory parameters subsequently improve, then this can become an intermittent, indefinite approach, at least until it appears that there is stability in the test results after ozone injections have been discontinued.

A tonsillectomy in an adult can be an arduous experience and should not be the first course of ac-

tion. But when a disease such as coronary atherosclerosis continues to worsen after all the other
prominent oral cavity infections have been effectively addressed and all other remediation efforts
have failed to produce a positive impact on laboratory tests or the clinical stability of the patient, a tonsillectomy can literally be life saving.

Conclusion

Focal infections in the oral cavity cause and
aggravate nearly all known chronic degenerative
diseases. Coronary heart disease and breast cancer are the conditions most consistently caused and
fed by these infections. Diagnosis must be pursued
even when there is no symptomatology referable to
the oral cavity. Once identified, a definitive therapy should be defined and executed. As emphasized
throughout this book, 3D cone beam imaging must
become part of the ***initial*** ***and*** ***routine follow-up***
evaluation of anyone with any significant chronic
disease, and even of the evaluation of the younger
person seeking a "well-person" workup for the first
time.

General Treatment Protocol for Chronic Degenerative Disease

Overview

A chronic degenerative disease refers to any disease in which there is a deterioration or break-down of structure and/or function of the involved tissue. As such, there really is no chronic disease that cannot be effectively categorized as a chronic degenerative disease. Of course, the two most prominent and impactful such diseases are atherosclerosis of the coronary arteries leading to heart attack and the malignant transformation of diseased tissues. Collectively, these two diseases claim the vast majority of lives in the United States and the other developed countries around the world today. However, the basic pathophysiological abnormalities seen in coronary heart disease and cancer are also seen in all of the other chronic degenerative diseases, including arthritis, autoimmune disease, hypertension, diabetes, and dementia, to name but a few.

As discussed earlier in some detail (particularly in Chapter 4), all diseases in the body are caused by increased oxidative stress, both intracellularly and extracellularly. Increased oxidative stress is nothing more than the presence of an abnormally high percentage of oxidized (electron-depleted) biomolecules in the affected organs, tissues, or other diseased areas of the body. Depending on the biomolecule, this state of oxidization results in that biomolecule having lost part or all of its normal chemical or biological function. However, when chemical reduction of that biomolecule occurs, with a restoration of the full complement of electrons, that biomolecule once again has normal chemical/ biological function.

Also, all abnormal oxidation of biomolecules in the body occurs because of the presence of toxins, all of which are either pro-oxidant in nature or directly resulting in a pro-oxidant effect. No disease or the symptoms of a disease can occur in the absence of an increased oxidation of biomolecules. These toxins are only countered effectively by nutrient biomolecules, which are chemically antioxidant, or electron-donating, in nature. All diseases feature an ongoing tug-of-war between pro-oxidants, or toxins, and nutrients, or antioxidants.

This continuing biomolecular war between electron depletion and electron repletion in all diseased tissues and organs requires a two-pronged approach to the treatment of any disease. These basic strategies or principles must always be kept in mind in putting together an optimally effective treatment protocol for any patient with any chronic degenerative disease:

1. **Stop or minimize the generation of new toxins in the body and/or the exposure of the body to new toxins.**
2. **Neutralize and eliminate existing toxins in the diseased tissues and repair as much oxidative damage to biomolecules as possible.**

This continuing biomolecular war between electron depletion and electron repletion in all diseased tissues and organs requires a two-pronged approach to the treatment of any disease.

In other words, it is really just as important to ***prevent new tissue damage*** as it is to ***repair old tissue damage***. And while this would seem to be a very straightforward and logical approach to clinical medicine, it is very rarely followed.

Almost all of the clinical treatment protocols for any chronic degenerative disease, even those that are generally regarded as the most effective, only address the repair of previously damaged tissue. It is generally assumed that degenerative disease is a matter of genetics, age, and/or lifestyle choices. Therefore, those designing treatment protocols appear to be generally unaware that ongoing toxin exposures both initiate and propagate cell/tissue damage. If I were to assume that my car tire is leaking air because it is old, or a cheaply made, I might resort to filling it with air every day. I probably wouldn't look for a nail, remove it, and repair the hole. But close attention to filling it with air could keep it going a long time.

But a failure to stop or minimize the generation of new toxins (the 1st principle) misses the best chances for long-term recovery.

Admittedly, eliminating or neutralizing existing toxins (the 2nd principle in the treatment of chronic degenerative disease) will often produce a noticeable benefit and even substantial clinical recovery. But a failure to stop or minimize the generation of new toxins (the 1st principle) misses the best chances for long-term recovery. It cannot be overemphasized, however, that addressing either or both of these two basic principles for treating chronic degenerative disease is **_vastly_ _superior_** to the primary goal of most of the mainstream medicine treatment protocols. Generally, the goal of such protocols is just to treat the symptoms of the disease as effectively as possible, leaving the underlying cause(s) of the disease completely unaddressed. The disease then continues its progressive tissue degeneration while symptoms are alleviated to a greater or lesser degree.

Basic Disease Treatment Principles

The effective treatment of any disease, then, depends on restoring and maintaining an optimal reduction/oxidation (redox) balance in the body. While the goal of minimizing oxidative stress throughout the body is simple and straightforward, accomplishing this goal is involved and requires attention to detail. The physiology and pathophysiology of the metabolic processes throughout the body are complex, and the response to an intervention in one individual does not guarantee the same response in another individual.

The effective treatment of any disease, then, depends on restoring and maintaining an optimal reduction/ oxidation (redox) balance in the body.

The clinician must regularly evaluate the clinical and laboratory responses of a patient to a given intervention to make sure that any untoward responses do not go undetected and unchecked. New pathologies, often in the form of new oral cavity focal infections, consistently develop over time, and a normal slate of clinical and laboratory results at one point in time is no assurance that the same normalcy will be present a year or two later. ***Quality follow-up evaluation is always essential for optimal care***.

Treatment principles for any chronic degenerative disease should always include the following:

1. Minimize new toxin exposure
2. Eliminate accumulated toxins
3. Identify and eradicate infections, especially chronic, silent ones
4. Attempt to normalize depressed levels of critical regulatory hormones, especially thyroid and sex
5. Optimize antioxidant and nutrient levels, especially vitamin C, throughout the body
6. Selectively and appropriately use prescription medicines

These treatment principles have been addressed earlier in this book, and to even a greater degree in previous books.[1-7] The essentials of each point will only be recapped here.

Minimize New Toxin Exposure

This is really the main point of this book. For most adults around the world, the pathogens and toxins coming from oral/dental infections cause many chronic degenerative diseases. Furthermore, they worsen all chronic degenerative diseases via the maintenance of a body-wide state of increased inflammation (increased oxidative stress).

Other significant sources of new toxins are inappropriate supplementation (calcium, iron, and copper), identifiable and avoidable environmental toxins (air, food, and water). New toxins in many adults also result from chronically poor digestion, with chronic food putrefaction and gut-derived pathogens and toxins.

New toxin exposure can also result when relatively inactive toxins from earlier exposure are mobilized from storage sites in the course of intentional or inadvertent detoxification measures. New toxins are also generated when pathogens and/or cancer cells are killed off.

Eliminate Accumulated Toxins

When toxins are mobilized from sites of accumulation or storage, they can exert renewed toxic effects unless they are strongly bound by a chelator until they are finally excreted. And even the best chelators have a certain degree of spontaneous dissociation from the substance to which they are bound.

When toxins are mobilized from sites of accumulation or storage, they can exert renewed toxic effects unless they are strongly bound by a chelator until they are finally excreted.

Some agents have only the ability to mobilize toxins but have no ability to bind the toxins after they are mobilized. Such agents need to be accompanied by a significant amount of antioxidants in supplemental or nutrient form in order for the toxin-mobilizing process to be achieved without negative clinical impact or clinical deterioration of the patient.

Common prescription chelators include dimercaptosuccinic acid (DMSA), dimercaptopropane sulfonate (DMPS), dimercaprol (BAL), ethylenediaminetetraacetic acid (EDTA), penicillamine, deferoxamine, and deferasirox. Effective nutrient chelators include alpha lipoic acid (ALA) and inositol hexaphosphate (IP6). Other supplements that work to stimulate natural chelation via glutathione and glutathione-related enzymes include whey protein, N-acetylcysteine, S-acetyl glutathione, and liposome-encapsulated glutathione. An excellent way to induce a broad-spectrum detoxification, with only a relatively minimal induction of detoxification side effects, is with induced sweating, especially when utilizing a far infrared sauna.

Identification and Eradication of Chronic Infections

Generally, focal infections are not clinically obvious, as has been extensively documented in this book. When an individual has any significant chronic degenerative disease, the oral cavity should be completely evaluated first. The teeth and sinuses should always be thoroughly evaluated with 3D cone beam imaging, even if thorough regular X-ray examinations reveal no clear pathology. When there is an increased level of suspicion, a variety of tests can be employed to look for chronic tonsillar infections, including direct pressure on physical examination, magnetic resonance imaging, computed tomography, transoral sonography, and optical coherence tomography with autofluorescence imaging.

Imaging techniques can also be used for not only tonsillar infection, but also for focal infections that are present throughout the body. This is of particular importance when either no oral cavity infections have been identified, or if such infections have been identified and eradicated, and significant clinical improvement is not then seen. These include PET scanning, gallium 67 scintigraphy, and scanning techniques utilizing labeled leukocytes, immunoglobulins, monoclonal antibodies, cytokines, liposomes, and peptides.

Employing any of a number of ozone applications, along with high-dose vitamin C and other antioxidants, is often very effective.

The eradication of identified focal infections depends on multiple factors, including the patient's desires and the tools with which the dentist and/or physician is familiar and comfortable. Employing any of a number of ozone applications, along with high-dose vitamin C and other antioxidants, is often very effective. The physical removal of infection and infected tissue, as with debridement or tooth extraction, is always the most direct way to effectively deal with a focal infection when feasible.

Correct Critical Hormone Deficiencies

Thyroid hormone deficiency and sex hormone deficiencies are very common, and they become more prevalent and more pronounced as aging proceeds. Much of what is accepted as the inevitable circumstances of "old age" is easily prevented or at least substantially attenuated with proper hormone replacement therapy. In general, especially with older individuals, bioidentical sex hormone replacement is the best option, and as a rule of thumb, replacement should not be initiated unless blood levels are objectively below normal, not just in the low portion of the reference range. Target levels should not exceed the middle of the reference range.

Thyroid hormone replacement should be adjusted by normalizing the T3/reverse T3 ratio, which reflects normal intracellular thyroid function.

Thyroid hormone replacement should be adjusted by normalizing the T3/reverse T3 ratio, which reflects normal intracellular thyroid function.

Normalization of both sex hormone and thyroid hormone levels functions to decrease body-wide oxidative stress, decrease systemic inflammation, and to decrease all-cause mortality. Much of this effect stems from the ability of normal thyroid and sex hormone levels to prevent the ability of focal infections to spread and take seed elsewhere, such as in the lining of the coronary arteries.

Optimize Antioxidant/Nutrient Levels

It should be logical that any protocol that strives to optimize antioxidants and antioxidant nutrients needs to include both minimizing the factors that consume antioxidants (toxins) as well as supplementing as completely as possible those antioxidant agents themselves. While there are literally hundreds of quality supplements available, it is obviously not feasible to take all of them. What they all share is the ability to fortify the quality and the quantity of the protective antioxidant matrix throughout the body.

There are also patient limitations, most notably: finances, the ability to stick to an involved regimen of supplementation, and the ability of the stomach to tolerate varying doses of multiple supplements without undue stomach upset. With these concepts in mind, then, it is generally advisable that any basic supplement regimen include as many of the following antioxidants and antioxidant nutrients as is feasible on a regular basis. Specific dosages are not being recommended due to the widely variable needs of different individuals with different diseases and differing daily toxin exposures.

Vitamin C, magnesium, vitamin K (including K2) and vitamin D3 are arguably the four most important and foundational supplements. It is inadvisable to avoid including any of these supplements in any long-term supplementation protocol. The supplementation of each of these agents individually is associated with a decrease in all-cause mortality,[8-13] meaning that they positively impact all diseased cells in the body. While these four supplements certainly have more than one biochemical function, they all work to help decrease intracellular levels of calcium and to normalize calcium metabolism throughout the body. As increased intracellular levels of calcium are always involved in the cells of any affected tissue becoming chronically diseased, it is very likely that the ability of these agents to help regulate calcium homeostasis in the body is the major reason why they are able to decrease the chances of dying from any disease or medical condition.

Other important supplements include mixed tocopherols (vitamin E source), beta carotene

> *Vitamin C, magnesium, vitamin K (including K2) and vitamin D3 are arguably the four most important and foundational supplements.*

(vitamin A source), the B vitamin Complex, lysine, proline, omega-3 fish oil (EPA and DHA source), and iodine/potassium iodide. A broad combination of amino acids is a good supplement as well. Other good supplements include coenzyme Q-10, N-acetyl cysteine, alpha lipoic acid, curcumin, MSM, aloe vera, and whey protein.

As long as calcium, copper, and iron supplementation are completely avoided, taking a multi-mineral supplement is a good idea for most individuals. However, some minerals can accumulate to toxic levels, so it is generally best to take the low end of the recommended dosing. Testing for individual mineral levels can help with adjusting the dosages of such a supplement over time, best done with the assistance of your chosen health care practitioner.

Too many well-meaning health care practitioners and their well-educated patients regard all pharmaceutical agents as something to be avoided.

Appropriate Use of Prescription Medicines

While modern medicine usually makes a habit of only treating symptoms while leaving the underlying disease process unchecked, some of the prescription medicines available do offer enormous benefits for both quality and length of life. Too many well-meaning health care practitioners and their well-educated patients regard all pharmaceutical agents as something to be avoided. While trying to be as well informed as possible is certainly appropriate, it does not mean that all drugs or remedies offered by Big Pharma and most doctors are automatically bad for you.

Ozone and
Oral Focal Infections

Overview

The oral cavity is a thriving microbial ecosystem. It serves as host to colonies of
normal microbes as well as an array of pathogenic microbes. This ecosystem, modulated to a
great degree by the health of the host's immune
defenses, works to keep the pathogenic microbe
population at a minimum. When circumstances
disturb the delicate balance however, these oppor-
tunistic pathogens can thrive and proliferate until
they establish a focal infection. As demonstrated in
Part One of this book, it is these focal infections that
initiate and sustain the majority of degenerative
diseases that plague mankind.

Many of these different pathogens are able to
resist removal or modulation by forming biofilms
(such as dental plaque) that play a large role in how
readily dental caries and periodontal disease take
hold. Eventually, this can lead to all of the other
focal dental infections/pathologies. Traditional

periodontal hygiene/infection protocols have been directed at mechanically removing periodontal biofilms along with the use of antibiotic therapy. This conventional approach to oral biofilms and other chronic oral infections is currently being augmented by a growing number of therapeutic ozone protocols.

These ozone applications have reliably resolved infections, accelerated healing, and even stimulated healthy bone growth where needed.

These ozone applications have reliably resolved infections, accelerated healing, and even stimulated healthy bone growth where needed. The demonstrated efficacy of ozone therapies should make the use of this agent mandatory in the practice of modern dentistry.

This chapter is not intended to be a comprehensive review of the biochemistry and biological applications of ozone. Rather, it aims to introduce the reader to the role of ozone as a valuable part of most medical therapeutic protocols, with particular attention to its important and multi-faceted applications for focal infections of the oral cavity.

Ozone Biochemistry Basics

Ozone has been used with great efficacy in Europe for over 150 years, especially in Germany and in Russia. In the United States, however, ozone's recognition as a therapeutic agent with its wide array of positive physiological effects is relatively recent. Nevertheless, its growing use in dental and medical applications in the U.S. has increased exponentially in the last two decades.[1]

The ozone molecules are composed of three oxygen atoms, while regular oxygen gas molecules are composed of two oxygen atoms. While oxygen gas is very stable, ozone gas is not, having a half-life of roughly 40 minutes. Although not technically a free radical, ozone has potent pro-oxidant properties, and it is very effective as a broad-spectrum antimicrobial agent. Also, ozone can be regarded as a crucial physiological activator.[2]

It is very important to realize that in many applications, ozone has positive clinical effects at one dosage and negative clinical effects at another dosage.

However, it is very important to realize that in many applications, ozone has positive clinical effects at one dosage and negative clinical effects at another dosage.[3,4] The point to take away from this is simple:

Use the recommended dosages of ozone in any given application that have withstood the test of time and proven themselves to be consistently beneficial.

Dosages outside of these recommended amounts should really only be employed in the context of ongoing research to see if new applications and new recommended dosages of ozone can be developed.

NEVER just assume that if a little ozone is good, more is better, or that a more concentrated or a more rapid application is better.

Ozone can be highly pro-oxidant in one application while at another dosage, often lower, it can stimulate intracellular pathways that actually produce a strong antioxidant effect. Depending on what is being treated, a strong to minimal pro-oxidant effect may be desirable, whereas in another clinical situation, a strong to minimal antioxidant effect may be desirable. The current recommendations for the many clinical applications of ozone have largely evolved over a very long period of time with many millions of administrations. These protocols have been developed via trial-and-error as to what works best, or by transitioning from effective dosing administrations in animal studies to similar dosing protocols in humans.

This methodical testing combined with an enormous number of trials has produced an ***incredible safety record of ozone when used as recommended***. What's more, these time-tested protocols deliver a clearly positive clinical impact in virtually every recommended application.

Conceptually, it is important to realize that ozone treatments on the blood generally induce only a fleeting pro-oxidant effect that is promptly neutralized by the predominant antioxidant capacity that is present. However, ozone metabolites are formed that exert ongoing biological and messenger effects on different biomolecules. Some of the most important of these metabolites occur when ozone reacts with cell membrane lipids to produce peroxides known as ozonides. And while the presence of ozone in the blood dissipates quickly, ozonides are stable for days to weeks and can easily penetrate cell membranes and exhibit selective oxidative properties. Also, ozonides oxidize NADH to NAD, which both produces oxygen and helps to normalize cellular energy metabolism.[5,6]

Ozone has been shown to have multiple documented positive physiological and biological effects, including the following:

- ✓ The activation of glycolysis in red blood cells resulting in increased ATP levels and improved oxygen release.[7] This effect occurs with either the mixing of ozone gas with the blood of the patient (autohemotherapy) or just the rectal insufflation of ozone gas. It has been suggested that these treated red blood

cells become "super-gifted erythrocytes" that can increase oxygen delivery
in hypoxic tissues and restore a normal
oxygen level, positively impacting many
diseases, including cancer.[8]

✓ A stimulatory effect on human natural
killer cells[9]

✓ A stimulatory effect on the release
of nitric oxide from endothelial cells,
helping in smooth muscle relaxation[10]

✓ Helps resolve or improve multiple clinical conditions,[11-13] including:

▸ Acute and chronic bacterial, viral, and
fungal infections

▸ Vascular disorders, especially
involving ischemia

▸ Disorders of immune depression/
suppression, activating T and B
lymphocytes, increasing immuno-
globulin synthesis, and enhancing
phagocytosis

▸ Chronic degenerative diseases,
including cardiac disease, cancer, and
neurodegenerative diseases, involving
the upregulation of antioxidant
enzyme capacity

▸ Orthopedic pathology, with pain alleviation and bone regeneration

▸ Wound healing

✓ Helps resolve or improve multiple dental pathologies, including:

- ▶ Bacterial pathogens and associated biofilms
- ▶ Periodontitis-related inflammation and infection
- ▶ Prevention of dental caries
- ▶ Remineralization of existing caries
- ▶ Tooth sensitivity
- ▶ Accelerated healing and tissue regeneration
- ▶ Teeth whitening
- ▶ Pathogen burden associated with root canal-treated teeth and other infected teeth; improved, faster healing with less pain and better infection control when infected teeth are extracted
- ▶ Bone regeneration in cavitations and tooth sockets
- ▶ Temporomandibular joint treatment
- ▶ Tonsil infection treatment

Ozone has many different ways in which it can be applied and utilized therapeutically. When it is immediately mixed into blood withdrawn from a patient, as in major autohemotherapy, the initial pro-oxidant effect is fleeting, and the dominant therapeutic effects are provided by the formation of ozonides that do not degrade rapidly. Also, depending on the dose and concentration of ozone given, there can also be a variable degree of upregulation of antioxidant enzymes inside the cells of the body.

Important: Unadulterated ozone gas that is directly inhaled is never indicated and always toxic.

Some of the many ways in which ozone has been successfully applied therapeutically include the following:

- ✓ Major and minor autohemotherapy
- ✓ Direct venous or intra-arterial injection (no longer recommended due to complications when technique is not performed correctly)
- ✓ Direct soft tissue/subcutaneous/intra-dermal injection
- ✓ Rinsing with or drinking ozonated water
- ✓ Application of ozonated olive oil
- ✓ Intramuscular injection
- ✓ Intra-articular (joint) injection
- ✓ Ambient gas application (bagging) or low-pressure application
- ✓ Ozone gas in body cavities (e.g., rectal, vaginal)
- ✓ Infusion of ozonated physiological saline[14]

Dental and Oral Cavity Ozone Applications

The applications to be addressed will just be those applied in the oral cavity that directly relate to the focal infections discussed in this book, rather than all dental applications in general. The main benefits of ozone in dealing with such infections are due to its ability to quickly and efficiently kill pathogens, to accelerate wound healing, and to promote the regeneration of bone, even in areas with persistent infection and tissue necrosis. Much of the following ozone application and dosage information comes the work of Philip Mollica, MS, DMD, NMD and Robert Harris, DMD, NMD.

...incorporating ozone in the treatment plan is going to produce better results in both the short- and long-term.

Regardless of whether extraction or an alternative treatment approach to an infected tooth is planned, incorporating ozone in the treatment plan is going to produce better results in both the short- and long-term. Where the general health of the patient has been compromised, collaboration between dentist and physician is essential – the more the better. Especially in advanced cancer and coronary heart disease, the proper extraction of infected teeth remains the optimal approach to give the patient the best chances of clinical stabilization or even complete recovery.

In such situations, ozone has proven to be so effective in promoting good healing in and around infected bone that approaches never considered as viable alternatives in the past can now be utilized. Some of those treatment approaches are itemized below. Such protocols should always include a meticulous monitoring and follow-up of basic blood work to help determine that the root canal-treated tooth or the untreated infected tooth with CAP is not having a significant negative impact on the general health. Probably the most important tests to monitor closely are C-reactive protein (CRP), glucose, cholesterol, LDL, HDL, and triglycerides (parameters of metabolic syndrome). Also important are the T3 and reverse T3 levels, along with sex hormone levels.

Probably the most important tests to monitor closely are C-reactive protein (CRP), glucose, cholesterol, LDL, HDL, and triglycerides...

Additional important tests would include any test that reflects increased body-wide inflammation, along with cancer biomarkers where appropriate. Serial nuclear imaging tests will be indicated in some patients. It is always advisable to start at the lowest recommended ozone concentrations and frequencies of treatment and increase gradually.

General ozone protocol principles to be applied for dental infections include the following:

1. **Asymptomatic CAP tooth**. Options include extraction and healing, extraction with immediate dental implant, extraction with delayed dental implant, and root canal treatment. Ozone gas, ranging from 40 to 60 micrograms/ml is injected ("fumigated") continuously into all evacuated root canal spaces over a 60-second period in the course of the root canal procedure. When an infected tooth is extracted, ozone gas ranging from 14 to 20 micrograms/ml with a 30 gauge needle is injected into the bony periapical area following debridement. Periodic repeat periapical injections can be performed to further facilitate and maintain good healing.

2. **Tooth previously root canal-treated**. As above, ozone injection can be done to try to stabilize a "failing" root canal that is developing increased CAP over time. Occasionally, the ozone treatment will stabilize the tooth. Sometimes, however, when the root canal procedure was not done with sufficient expertise, a repeat root canal procedure might be indicated to get a better pulpal seal, allowing a

lessening and even resolution of the CAP at the apex. In general, however, if a good seal was not obtained with the initial root canal procedure, the patient should not be subjected to a repeat procedure and a minimum of months of needless pathogen/toxin exposure. It is very important that clear improvement of abnormal lab tests accompany such interventions, or there will be a much greater urgency in advising the patient to proceed to extraction. Also, a worsening of lab tests will even further increase the urgency for extraction. As above, repeat periapical injections can be performed to further facilitate good healing, and to possibly stabilize the infected tooth.

3. **Chronic periodontal disease**. Effective ozone approaches include irrigating periodontal pockets with ozonated water and by injecting gas ("insufflation") in those same pockets, concentration 20 to 30 micrograms/ml. Follow-up treatments (healing/supportive phase versus infective phase) should use ozone concentrations between 6 and 10 micrograms/ml. Repeated applications of ozonated olive oil to these gum areas can be continued at home.

4. **Peri-implant mucositis and peri-implantitis**. The ozone approach to these conditions would include the periapical injections described in category 1 noted above, along with the ozone approach for chronic periodontal disease also noted above.

5. **Suspected chronic tonsillar infection**. Ozone gas at a concentration of 15 to 20 micrograms/ml, volume 2.5 cc per tonsil, is injected with a 30 gauge needle. Four to five injection sessions over a few months is usually advisable (Madrid Declaration on Ozone Therapy, approved 2010) for optimal healing. It is very important to include follow-up with blood work that reflects increased oxidative stress in the body as to whether a positive systemic effect is being seen, as would be the case when the CRP level decreases. In Cuban patients with tonsillitis, the ozone dose was pushed to 50 micrograms/ml, with 5 cc in each tonsil, in a series of 2,300 patients, for a total of four sessions. Laboratory parameters of increased oxidative stress were followed in some of the patients and found to decline after the injections. A "success" rate of 97% was seen, and surgical intervention was avoided.

6. **Cavitational osteonecrosis**. For a "simple" cavitation that is relatively small and well-contained, ozone injections can be made directly inside the cavitation, as well as around the bony lower periphery of the site, usually in the dosage described above for periapical injections. When the cavitation is large and appearing to grow over time, a larger area of bone can be injected as felt necessary. Repeat injections are nearly always advisable to get the best long-term outcome, which would include the regeneration of new bone around and even inside the cavitation. Ozone can be effective in regenerating significant amounts of bone even when cavitations have been large and dormant, or even growing, for decades.

7. **Chronic oral cavity infections and pathogen colonizations**. Nasal insufflation is an application that helps to normalize the oral cavity and nasopharyngeal microbial flora, giving good support to the maintenance of positive outcomes following the treatment of any the oral cavity focal infections described above. It can also rapidly accelerate the resolution of colds, cough, and influenza. Ozone is bubbled through

olive oil at a flow rate of ½ liter/minute with a concentration of 25 to 30 micrograms/ml, and normal inhalation via a nasal cannula can proceed for 25 to 30 minutes per session. Remember that ozone is very toxic when inhaled directly. However, the ozone forms an ozonide after bubbling through the olive oil that is well-tolerated and not directly pro-oxidant in nature. An oxidant effect is only realized later when the ozonide dissolves in an aqueous environment.

8. **Chronic sinusitis**. Nasal insufflations, as noted above, help to resolve chronic sinusitis, particularly when there is not an inflamed or infected upper jawbone tooth chronically feeding the sinus inflammation/infection. In addition to the nasal insufflation technique, 12 ml of ozone at a concentration of 20 micrograms/ml can be drawn up into a syringe and slowly injected into a nostril, usually facilitated with a tubular extension on the end of the syringe, while breathing through the mouth. This can then be repeated for the other nostril. There should be no respiratory irritation or cough if done correctly.

There are certainly multiple other ways to administer ozone to the oral cavity and other areas of the body, depending on the medical condition and whether infection eradication is the goal, or maintenance of an uninfected state is desired, or when infection containment and stabilization is desired. Specific dental protocols for dealing with infected gums and teeth vary widely in detail, and there is still no one acknowledged perfect approach yet established for a given dental application.

Conclusion

The oral cavity is clearly the primary site of the most clinically impactful focal infections and sources of body-wide increased oxidative stress. Therefore, it is essential that dental protocols are optimally efficient in controlling and, if possible, completely eradicating such infections whenever and wherever they are encountered. Properly applied ozone for such oral cavity infections is proving to be one of the most important and effective tools in achieving this goal and optimizing both oral and general health.

Integrative Patient Care
and
Informed Consent

Overview

A patient is best served when all healthcare practitioners involved in the care of that patient actively interact and exchange pertinent information regarding evaluation, treatment, and ongoing follow-up. General practitioners and internists routinely share patient information with specialists such as cardiologists, neurosurgeons, and endocrinologists, because of the obvious connections between the respective parts of the body each specialist treats and the patient's overall health.

With regard to dentists and physicians, this integration of disciplines remains almost completely absent. Generally, there is agreement that an acutely infected, very painful tooth can have serious ramifications to the general health of a patient if left unaddressed. Beyond that, however, medical practitioners and dentists both function as if the mouth and the body were totally separate and unconnected entities. In essence, it is accepted that dental problems are limited to the domain of the mouth, while heart disease, cancer, and other chronic diseases are in the exclusive domain of the non-oral portions of the body.

The overwhelming body of data from these studies makes it very clear that pathology in the mouth is intimately interrelated with pathology throughout the rest of the body.

Aside from the obvious reality that the mouth and body share the same cardiovascular system, endocrine system, lymphatic system, digestive system, and nervous system, there is even more compelling evidence of their interconnectedness with regard to health and disease. The studies in this book come from the peer-reviewed scientific literature in both the dental and medical arenas. The overwhelming body of data from these studies makes it very clear that pathology in the mouth is intimately interrelated with pathology throughout the rest of the body. Furthermore, those studies also show that such oral pathology, in the form of clinically silent infections, is the **_primary_** reason for the initiation and evolution of many, if not most, chronic diseases.

A further aspect of such complete integrative patient care involves a complete informed consent before any procedure is performed on the patient. Dentists need to be aware of established medical consequences to a dental procedure in the same manner that physicians need to know that dental evaluation, and potentially needed dental treatment, is at the top of the list of considerations for any patients with newly-diagnosed conditions, especially coronary heart disease and breast cancer. And before any patient gives consent to any procedure, that patient needs to be optimally informed on this mouth-disease connection as well.

Coordinated Health Care

The almost total segregation between medicine and dentistry begins at the basic educational level. There is no integration of the two disciplines in either medical school or dental school. In addition, at the time of this writing, there are no significant continuing education conferences in mainstream dentistry or medicine that address the essential connections between these two disciplines once dentists and physicians are in private practice or pursuing academic careers. In the realm of integrative (aka complementary, holistic, biological, and/or alternative) dentistry

And before any patient gives consent to any procedure, that patient needs to be optimally informed on this mouth-disease connection as well.

and medicine, a few conferences are finally starting to address the important dentistry-medicine connections.

The optimal way to bring needed integration between these disciplines would be to incorporate dental schools into medical schools. A student interested in dentistry would be trained in the same way as any medical student, ultimately specializing in the practice of dental medicine. These students would perform rotations in internal medicine in addition to rotations in dental offices. Similarly, and just as importantly, medical students would have to have rotations in dental offices. In this way all graduating physicians, regardless of specialty, would understand the vital connection between the medical and dental disciplines from the outset of their formal training. A similar integration of dentistry and medicine could also occur in the rotations during internship and residency programs.

No dental patient should ever receive any kind of dental procedure without having certain baseline blood testing and diagnostic evaluation.

For the Dentist

No dental patient should ever receive any kind of dental procedure without having certain baseline blood testing and diagnostic evaluation. If the patient has a physician and has had recent blood testing, this can be requested for review rather than be redone. While a wide variety of blood test results could be helpful, the following tests should always be done as a baseline prior to any dental work:

1. CBC and biochemistry panel, which should include a lipid panel
2. C-reactive protein, high sensitivity (hs-CRP)

As discussed previously, these tests are of paramount importance since they test the parameters that track metabolic syndrome, the results of which reliably worsen if coronary artery disease develops and is continuing to evolve. Also, the CRP level is extremely important as a baseline test to know how a future dental infection might be impacting body-wide health. When glucose, lipids, and CRP are all clearly outside of the reference range, a high index of suspicion for oral cavity infections should be present. This is especially important if the patient is younger and does not yet have any established chronic degenerative disease diagnoses, and appropriate interventions can prevent significant chronic diseases from getting established.

When glucose, lipids, and CRP are all clearly outside of the reference range, a high index of suspicion for oral cavity infections should be present.

If financially feasible for the patient, baseline 3D cone beam imaging should be done to either immediately identify evolving dental pathology, or to establish as a baseline that the patient does not yet have any chronically infected teeth. However, if the laboratory testing noted above is clearly abnormal, the 3D cone beam imaging should **always** be performed in the best interests of the patient.

> *...if the laboratory testing noted above is clearly abnormal, the 3D cone beam imaging should **always** be performed in the best interests of the patient.*

Whenever 3D cone beam imaging is performed, the images should be interpreted by an interventional radiologist and/or dentist with established expertise in such interpretation. It should always be reported on the procedure request form that a search for CAP of any degree is a primary goal of the procedure. Any diagnostic procedure is greatly augmented in the yield of meaningful information when the interpreter has substantial experience AND as much information is provided to the interpreter as to the reason for the examination. When an interpreter knows the concerns of the ordering dentist/physician, the amount and quality of the information gleaned from 3D X-ray, or any other diagnostic study, is often greatly enhanced.

It should also be routine for all dental offices to take blood pressure and pulse measurements. As a general rule of thumb, if the patient has a persistent diastolic blood pressure above 100 and/or a persistent pulse rate above 100, strong consideration should be given to delaying the dental work until the patient has been evaluated and cleared for treatment by a physician. Admittedly, some situations justify immediate dental intervention—as when the patient is presenting with an acutely abscessed and painful tooth. In this case, the high blood pressure and elevated heart rate might be largely due to the infected tooth.

For the Physician

The primary care physician should ***always*** consider the possibility of occult oral cavity infections as a contributing etiological factor in any patient with a chronic degenerative disease. This is especially the case when the CRP and lipid blood tests are significantly abnormal. Granted, at the time of the writing of this book, a referral from the physician to the dentist for baseline evaluation, which would include 3D cone beam imaging of the teeth, does not occur. But the weight of information in this book mandates

> *The primary care physician should **always** consider the possibility of occult oral cavity infections as a contributing etiological factor in any patient with a chronic degenerative disease.*

that such referrals become routine. For the patient to receive optimal acute and long-term care, this **must** become the standard of care. Currently, no dentist or physician is in serious danger of having a malpractice suit stick for not looking at the critical connection between oral infections and chronic disease. However, medical/dental literature that reinforces the significance and prevalence of this connection continues to mount.

...the day will come when a cardiologist will be successfully sued by coronary heart disease patients...because no effort was made to look for the culprit dental infections...

Eventually, the physician and the dentist will simply be expected to exert the due diligence needed to stay current on issues that can threaten the well-being of their patients. This point in time will be hastened in its arrival by motivated and highly intelligent patients who become increasingly aware of this information as they research their own health issues on the internet and in books like this. Furthermore, the day will come when a cardiologist will be successfully sued by coronary heart disease patients who sustained heart attacks or underwent unnecessary interventions like angioplasty and bypass surgery only because no effort was made to look for the culprit dental infections that are so commonly responsible for this arterial disease. Physicians and dentists alike are expected to stay current with the pertinent scientific literature. Eventually, the assertion that "No one else is working up patients this way" will no longer be a credible defense in a malpractice suit from a damaged patient or the family of a deceased patient. Similarly, when a dentist misses one or more CAP teeth because the 3D cone beam imaging was not part of the initial dental work-up and a heart attack ensues some time later, a charge of negligence and dental malpractice will eventually stick as well.

Fully Informed Consent

Informed consent for dental procedures is generally deficient. Especially in light of the articles in the current scientific literature, many of which have been cited in this book, it fails to adequately inform patients of potentially foreseeable poor outcomes. An exemplary informed consent form for a root canal procedure that is currently recommended

Informed consent for dental procedures is generally deficient.

by the International Academy of Oral Medicine and Toxicology (IAOMT) as of 2015 appears on the next page, with minor modifications pertinent to the information in this book.

It is also important to realize that a fully informed consent can protect the dentist as much or more than it helps the patient understand procedural risks and make a properly informed decision—especially when it is executed in a conscientious and appropriate manner. All dental and medical procedures can have poor outcomes, and short of clear negligence in a procedure not performed to the current standard of care, the dentist or physician should never be successfully sued just because a poor outcome resulted.

This protection can be optimized now that the technology of the smartphone is so widely available. Every dental office should have a designated space for executing the informed consent with the designated office staff having the patient read the form and ask any questions if any confusion exists or clarification is needed. A smartphone can make a video of the event, and the dentist can briefly appear just prior to the patient's signing of the consent to make sure no question goes unanswered. The video can then be placed in a computer file with the date and name of the patient.

Making a video of the informed consent will keep the majority of suits from ever being filed. The patient looking for a quick settlement after an undesirable outcome will be keenly aware of what was said and how it was explained. There will be no defense on the part of the patient of not having been properly informed on the nature of the procedure and the possibility of a poor outcome. Knowing such a video exists will prevent most such cases from proceeding forward, especially if the poor outcome cannot be attributed to poor surgical technique or defective protocol.

It is also vital that dentists make a concerted effort to be detailed and comprehensive in the documentation in the chart of all that takes place. Poor progress notes are often an Achilles' heel for greater legal exposure, even when everything was done correctly. Written documentation must always be thorough.

Conclusion

Dentists and physicians need to be routinely, not rarely, coordinated in rendering the best health care for their patients. In light of the now well-established connections, often cause-and-effect in nature, between oral infections and chronic disease, this coordination is mandatory. Dentists need to incorporate minimal blood testing and physical evaluation before proceeding with dental procedures, and physicians need to have a very low threshold for referring their patients to dentists for the evaluation of occult infections in the mouth.

Informed consents need to include information from the current scientific literature to optimally educate the patients as to the risks associated with the procedures they choose to undergo. Dental and medical malpractice suits can be expected to increase if the now-established oral infection-chronic disease connection remains unrecognized and never factors into being a vital part of the best treatment protocol for a given patient.

International Academy of Oral Medicine and Toxicology (IAOMT)

Informed Consent for Endodontic Procedure (Root Canal Treatment)

Procedure and Indications

Your dentist is offering you the option of having a root canal treatment on one or more of your teeth. A root canal will allow you to keep your natural tooth (teeth). The alternative option to a root canal procedure is tooth extraction. If extraction is the treatment of choice, treatment options for the missing space(s) include: no treatment, removable partial denture, fixed bridge, or a dental implant.

The usual reason for having a root canal procedure is infection or necrosis of the dental pulp with or without associated pain.

The root canal procedure itself involves gaining access through the top of the tooth in order to reach the inside core of the tooth, which contains the pulp tissue. After access is achieved, specialized instruments are used to progressively evacuate, widen, and shape this pulp space (also known as the root canal space) in order to remove as much infected pulp material as possible along with the blood vessels, connective tissue, and the pain-signaling nerve fibers. This is designed to result in a pain-free tooth by the end of the procedure.

Procedure Outcomes

Very many root canal procedures are performed every day around the world, and the procedure itself is generally very safe to undertake. Many individuals have this procedure and remain pain-free for many years. Others can end up having continued or recurrent pain, sometimes with renewed evidence of infection, and they can elect to have the root canal-treated tooth retreated with another root canal procedure, or they can then elect to have the tooth extracted. Extraction immediately followed by an implant procedure is also an option.

Possible Side Effects

In order to consent to this procedure, it is important to understand that controversy surrounds the long-term safety of this procedure. Many experts have polar opposite opinions on the benefits and risks of this procedure. Much of this difference stems from the idea that many dentists feel infection is either eliminated by the procedure or reduced to a clinically inconsequential level in the treated tooth. Others, however, feel that significant infection remains most or all of the time, even though a subjective symptom such as pain, or an objective finding such as apical pathology on X-Ray (CAP), is not present.

Recent scientific literature has shown that having one or more root canal procedures is associated with an increased incidence of coronary heart disease. Another recent (2013) study examined the blood clots that caused heart attacks (myocardial infarction) and found a high concentration of the DNA found in the pathogens most commonly seen in root canal-treated teeth, as well as in chronic gum disease, the vast majority of the time. The same types of oral pathogen DNA have also been identified in a majority of ruptured intracranial aneurysm specimens obtained from patients, as well as in a majority of the samples of pericardial fluid surrounding the hearts of chronic coronary artery disease patients.

The overall health of the body depends on many different factors, and it is not anticipated that a root canal treatment will negatively impact every person who receives this treatment. Many patients do well indefinitely with well-performed procedures, from a dental and general health point of view. However, many of these teeth stay in the patient for a very long time, and a chronic low-grade infection can potentially cause general health problems years down the road, not just days, weeks, or months after the procedure, whether inside a root canal-treated tooth or anywhere else in the body.

I have read this consent form to have one or more root canal procedures. All of my questions and concerns have been addressed to my satisfaction. I wish to proceed with this part of my dental treatment.

_____   _____
Signature   Date

_____
Print Name

_____   _____
Witness   Date

Book Overview with Practical Suggestions

The writing of this book involved digging deep into the medical/dental literature to find the most significant peer-reviewed studies supporting the important messages and conclusions in this book. For those individuals who are looking for answers to their health questions but are not quite up to diving into a large amount of scientific data as it relates to medical and dental pathophysiology, this appendix is being offered. And for those health care providers and motivated laypersons who want to understand all of the reasons why a scientific conclusion is being reached and/or a therapeutic suggestion is being offered, this appendix is available to address those issues as best as possible.

This brief overview, then, will give the reader all of the main assertions and conclusions that are developed throughout the book, along with the straightforward advice as to how to apply those conclusions in your own personal pursuit of optimal health in as straightforward a manner as is possible.

Important Basic Health/Disease Facts

1. Excess oxidation of the biomolecules in your body is the underlying reason for all disease.

2. Important biomolecules include enzymes, proteins, sugars, lipids, and nucleic acids.

3. When something is oxidized, it loses electrons (as with rusted metal).

4. Oxidation of a biomolecule diminishes its normal physiological function, or it can render it completely non-functional.

5. Oxidized biomolecules can be restored to a state of normal function by the process of reduction (receiving electrons from an antioxidant). An antioxidant is the most potent and effective antitoxin because of its ability to donate electrons to oxidized biomolecules and electron-depleted toxins. Donating electrons to toxins blocks their ability to inflict their toxic damage.

6. The degree to which your biomolecules are oxidized, and where they are located, determines what disease will manifest and the level of severity.

7. All toxins (or poisons) inflict their damage on the body by the degree to which they result in the oxidation of important biomolecules. When the biomolecules are immediately critical to the vital metabolism of cells, a toxin (like cyanide) can kill quickly. When biomolecules of lesser physiological importance are the targets of oxidation, mild symptoms along with any of the chronic diseases can develop and evolve over a more extended period of time.

8. The greatest sources of potent toxins come from areas of focal infection, typically worsened by an oxygen-deprived local microenvironment, as with infected teeth.

9. As long as a focal infection remains unresolved, toxins are continually produced 24/7, and the rest of the body is subjected to increasing cumulative oxidative stress (more biomolecules becoming oxidized and remaining oxidized).

10. All chronic diseases have increased oxidative stress inside the affected cells, and all cancer cells have even greater increases in intracellular oxidative stress than nonmalignant diseased cells.

11. Although focal infections are the most important sources of toxins and increased oxidative stress throughout the body, other sources of toxins can be very significant for any given patient.

12. Environmental toxin exposure (water, food, air) can be minimal to massive in degree.

13. Toxic supplementation is very significant for many people. The most significant toxic supplements are calcium, iron, and copper, which should never be supplemented. The only exception is the supplementation of iron for an iron deficiency anemia, and only for as long as it takes to restore a normal red blood cell count.

14. Enriched or fortified foods should be carefully avoided, as they are a continuous source of toxic iron supplementation, and over a prolonged period of intake a state of body-wide increased oxidative stress develops due to iron accumulation. Such foods also cause chronic digestive disorders, both initiating and sustaining a leaky gut syndrome. This sets the stage for developing and maintaining a wide variety of food allergies, including peanut- and

gluten-related, along with autoimmune diseases.

15. Pathogens in infections or areas of pathogen overgrowth are the greatest sources of potent toxins and increased oxidative stress in the body.

16. The most important focal infections that cause the most chronic disease, especially heart disease and cancer, are infected teeth, infected gums and infected tooth-supportive bone and tissue, jawbone cavitations, infected dental implants, infected tonsils, infected sinuses, and soft tissue infections of the head and neck.

17. Of much less statistical significance than those located in the oral cavity, focal infections can be present throughout the body. A variety of imaging studies can be done when there is a significant chronic disease, and no evidence of oral cavity focal infection is found and addressed first.

18. The negative systemic impact of focal infections can be lessened enormously, and even largely negated in many individuals, by the maintenance of normal sex hormone and thyroid hormone status.

19. Sex hormone (testosterone for men, estrogen for women) replacement should never have a target level of more than the mid-range of normal, except for younger individuals. Bioidentical hormone replacement is advisable whenever possible.

20. Thyroid replacement should be largely based on the ratio of T3 to reverse T3, not traditional thyroid tests, as this ratio reflects the intracellular thyroid status of the cells throughout the body and not necessarily of the thyroid gland itself. Even when the thyroid gland is functioning normally, it is the metabolism of T3 inside the cells of the body that determines whether someone has a clinically normal or hypothyroid status. Thyroid replacement should include T3, as T4 is often not effectively converted to T3 inside the cells. As T3 is the active form of thyroid hormone, there is often little significant clinical impact from T4 administration, since the T4 to T3 conversion is not proceeding normally intracellularly. A T3 to reverse T3 ratio should be at least 18 to 1 or higher.

Important Oral Cavity Focal Infections and Practical Considerations

1. Infected teeth, infected gums, and infected tonsils are the most important and statistically significant focal infections in the oral cavity, in terms of negative health impact.

2. The most common oral cavity focal infections are root canal-treated teeth.

3. A minimum of 50% and as many as 80% of adults around the world have at least one root canal-treated tooth.

4. 100% of root canal-treated teeth are chronically infected. However, the toxic impact of such a tooth is highly variable, depending on many factors, including how effectively the dentist sealed off the pulp when the procedure was done, whether sex hormone and thyroid hormone status is normal, and whether there is X-ray evidence of significant apical radiolucency (infection) immediately after the procedure and in long-term follow-up. Serial C-reactive protein levels are also very important in determining whether the infected tooth is resulting in an increase in body-wide inflammation.

5. Statistically speaking, having had a root canal procedure increases your chance of having a heart attack. However, some people with root canal-treated teeth do very well for years without appearing to have significant negative impact on their general health. Much more research is needed to better define ahead of time which root canal-treated teeth are going to cause the most significant health problems, following research patients with the factors listed above in item #4.

6. In addition to root canal-treated teeth, very many adults around the world also have chronically infected teeth that have never received a dental procedure (chronic apical periodontitis—CAP). These teeth usually are **_not_** painful, and the patient has no symptoms to cause any suspicion that a severely infected tooth is present in the mouth. These teeth cause and sustain very many different chronic diseases, especially heart disease and cancer, even more so than root canal-treated teeth.

7. An untreated CAP tooth is present in 5% to 10% of adults around the world.

8. CAP is also present in root canal-treated teeth as much as 90% of the time.

9. CAP, the ongoing manifestation of persistent infection in and around the apex of the tooth, is present in between 60% to 80% of all adults around the world, when including its persistent presence following root canal treatment.

10. This means that a chronic tooth infection is present in a substantial majority of all adults, and it is often never suspected of being present.

11. A substantial number of chronically infected teeth are never detected on regular X-ray examination. (See Appendix with 2D and 3D X-ray images on the same infected tooth.)

12. 3D cone beam imaging of the teeth is the new gold standard for detecting clinically silent infected teeth. It is much more sensitive and accurate than any X-ray or other form of imaging.

13. It is now clearly established that oral pathogens and toxins from infected teeth and gums ***directly*** ***cause*** at least 90% of all heart attacks.

14. It also appears that the same oral pathogens and toxins from infected teeth and gums cause the vast majority of cases of breast cancer.

15. Oral pathogens and toxins from infected teeth and gums have strong associations

and links with most of the most common chronic degenerative diseases. These pathogens feed an increase in oxidative stress throughout the body, and this increased oxidative stress is strongly linked with an increased all-cause mortality (death for any reason), but especially mortality secondary to heart disease and cancer.

16. One clinic for the treatment of advanced cancer patients found multiple, chronically infected teeth in **98%** of the patient population.

17. The same population of advanced cancer patients were also found to always have chronically infected tonsils.

18. Chronically infected tonsils nearly always result from a sustained exposure to chronically infected teeth, and the tonsillar infections do **not** resolve on their own after the infected teeth have been extracted or otherwise effectively addressed.

19. It appears that tracking serial C-reactive protein (CRP) levels is currently the best way to know whether a focal infection is well-contained and clinically inconsequential, or having anywhere from a minimal to a massive impact on general health. Following other laboratory

parameters of increased oxidative stress or inflammation throughout the body is similarly useful, but CRP levels have been studied the most.

20. A CRP level of 0.5 ng/ml or lower is the true "normal" for this test, not the reference range levels of 0 to 3.0 ng/ml. Progressively higher levels of CRP generally indicate that something is feeding body-wide oxidative stress to a progressively greater degree. Patients with widespread cancers often have very elevated CRP levels.

21. When CRP levels remain elevated after oral infections have been addressed, there are either more unidentified focal infections, or the treatment of the identified focal infections was not adequately effective (e.g., a root canal-treated tooth with persistent CAP).

22. When all oral cavity infections are felt to have been identified and properly addressed and the CRP remains elevated, a series of ozone gas injections directly into the tonsils should be done, even if the tonsils appear normal on physical examination. If CRP levels then drop, this indicates some degree of healing in those tonsils. This is also a reasonable intervention as a part of

the total protocol for treating/removing infected teeth.

23. Ozone should be used whenever possible in dental interventions to facilitate infection control/resolution, improved wound healing, and improved bone regeneration.

General Protocol for Chronic Degenerative Disease

1. General Treatment Principles
    ✓ Prevent/minimize new daily toxin exposure (dental, environmental, dietary, digestive).
    ✓ Neutralize existing toxins already present in the body.
    ✓ Excrete/eliminate toxins in as non-toxic a manner as possible.
    ✓ Resolve existing focal infections, and eliminate the reasons for contracting new infections.
    ✓ Supplement optimally to maximize the antioxidant/nutrient status in the body
    ✓ Eat and digest optimally to maximize the antioxidant/nutrient status in the body. Consider regularly using a complete food pulverization device such as a NutriBullet.

> ✓ Correct hormone imbalances, typically deficiencies of testosterone, estrogen, and thyroid hormone.
> ✓ Use prescription medicines sparingly and appropriately, when the measures above do not resolve or control a significant condition adequately (e.g., control of high blood pressure, angina, significant symptoms such as pain); long-acting calcium channel blockers are of particularly great benefit.

2. ***Always*** include 3D cone beam imaging of the teeth as part of the baseline workup for any chronic degenerative disease, especially heart disease and breast cancer, and repeat this examination periodically for the optimal long-term management of any medical condition.

3. Always include in the baseline laboratory evaluation of the patient a full hormone panel, a full thyroid panel with T3 and reverse T3 levels, CRP measurement (along with any other laboratory tests tracking inflammation that can be afforded), and repeat these tests periodically for the optimal long-term management of any medical condition

4. Have the oral surgeon, endodontist, or dentist follow a infected tooth extraction

protocol that completely removes the periodontal ligament and all infected bone, and that incorporates established measures to optimize good healing, including ozone applications and platelet-rich plasma. There is a suggested protocol at the end of the book.

5. Always attempt to have your physician communicate with your dentist in constructing your long-term healthcare management, and vice-versa.

6. Bearing in mind there are many quality supplements that offer clear health benefits, always include the following supplements in your daily regimen, if possible. Dosage ranges are only very general. For supplements without established toxic levels of intake, more can always be supplemented as desired and depending on clinical/laboratory responses.

Supplementation Guidelines

These <u>baseline</u> guidelines are very general and should be adjusted to meet individual circumstances and health considerations

Nutrient	General Daily Dose	Form	Considerations
Vitamin A	25,000 IU	As beta carotene	Can build up toxicity so stay within recommended dose ranges
Vitamin B	Up to product's recommended dose	Complete complex without iron, copper, calcium	Excess B vitamins not toxic but also not necessary
Vitamin C	2,000mg to 15,000mg in divided doses	Sodium ascorbate or ascorbic acid	No toxic range established, should be limited largely by bowel tolerence
Vitamin C	1,000mg to 2,000mg	Liposome-encapsulated	No toxic range established
Vitamin C	1,000mg to 2,000mg	Fat-soluble (ascorbyl palmitate)	Stay within recommended range
Vitamin D3	5,000 IU		Use blood testing to adjust dosage to stay roughly in a blood level range of 50 to 80 ng/ml over time
Vitamin E	800 IU	Mixed tocopherols	Can build up toxicity

Continued on Next Page

Supplementation Guidelines

(Continued from previous page)

Nutrient	General Daily Dose	Form	Considerations
Vitamin K	3mg to 6mg	Menaquinone-4 or menatetre-none	No toxic range established
Lysine	2,500mg	Should be taken together in 5 to 1 ratio	
Proline	500mg		
Magnesium	400mg to 1,000mg in divided doses limited largely by bowel tolerance	Chelated form (such as glycinate)	Can build up toxicity from IV, but not from oral dosing
Multi-mineral	Up to product's recommended dose	Without iron, copper and no to very limited cal-cium	Can build up toxicity
Omega 3 Fish Oil	1g to 6 g daily or as directed on bottle	With EPA and DHA content	Generally non-toxic
Iodine/ Potassium Iodine	12.5 to 25 mg daily	Tablet	Generally non-toxic

Surgical Protocol for Extractions of Infected Teeth and Cavitation Surgery

General Observations

Tooth extractions, especially of infected teeth like untreated teeth with chronic apical periodontitis (CAP) or teeth having received root canal treatments, and cavitation debridement are surgical procedures performed in the oral cavity that involve both the soft tissues of the mouth, such as the gingiva, and the bones of the maxilla and mandible. Strict adherence to surgical protocols, such as those practiced by orthopedic surgeons, should also apply to oral surgery procedures.

It must be remembered that dentists, as surgeons of the oral cavity, are still operating on bone. Although the mouth is a more forgiving place to operate in terms of the healing of soft tissue, infected bone is difficult to completely heal no matter where in the body it is located. With the inability to isolate and create a sterile field when operating in the mouth, the potential to develop a post-surgical infection in the jawbone is always a significant possibility.

Furthermore, the ability of the mouth to rapidly heal soft tissue infections tends to make many dentists feel that infected bone in the mouth will heal just as readily, which is not necessarily the case. We now know how easily cavitations develop, and the X-ray appearance of seemingly complete healing after many routine dental extractions remains an illusion. Accepted surgical procedures must be followed everywhere in the body in order to optimize the chances of complete healing and complete clinical recovery.

If some of the periodontal ligament remains in the tooth socket after an extraction, or there is a failure to remove all of the infection in the jawbone, the remaining hole in the jawbone may not completely fill in with new bone. This void in the jawbone is called a cavitation and by its very nature, it can be a breeding ground for the same bacteria that infected the tooth in the first place. Because they are often surrounded by intact jawbone with multiple "natural" defects, cavitations often escape X-ray detection.

Therefore, to optimize the chances of complete healing and complete clinical recovery, accepted surgical procedures must be followed everywhere in the body—and especially in the mouth.

Oral Surgery Protocol

1. A complete patient medical and dental history, including consultation with all treating physicians, is essential before treatment is rendered. As the mouth is not isolated from the rest of the body, such a complete history is important. Nearly all dental procedures, especially surgery, have systemic, body-wide effects.

2. A thorough dental evaluation of the hard and soft tissues of the oral cavity is essential. The examination should include all necessary X-rays, including 3D imaging, along with a complete clinical exam. This includes pulp vitality tests of the teeth to determine which teeth are healthy and alive and which teeth might be unexpectedly nerve-dead and non-vital. Any additional tests that may aid in diagnosis and treatment planning should also be performed. It is important to point out that pulp vitality tests are an integral part in assessing the health of the teeth that did not receive root canal treatments. A dead, non-vital tooth in the mouth can be just as serious as a root canal-treated tooth,

as is the case with the untreated CAP tooth.

3. After the initial assessment of the patient's condition, a treatment plan must be established. If the treatment plan includes extractions and/or cavitation surgery, it is important to seek a surgeon who is not only surgically skilled, but who also has the ability to deliver intravenous medicines. Intravenous sedation is often necessary, and there must also be an access for the administration of appropriate antibiotics. The ability to administer ozone in a number of different ways is also very important in facilitating infection resolution and rapid wound healing.

4. Alternative treatments involving the injection of various remedies like Sanum remedies into the site of infection, like the bone around a root canal-treated tooth or around other infected teeth, should not be done. Similarly, such injections should not be made into cavitation sites. Many of these treatments actually make the disease process worse. Furthermore, there are some dentists advocating the use of these medicaments instead of surgery. It is impossible to restore dead bone to live bone

again with any medication. Surgery must be performed to remove all of the dead and infected bone as well as establishing adequate perfusion of blood from adjacent healthy bone into the surgical site. This is the only way healing can occur. However, a wide variety of ozone applications, including injections in and around cavitations and infected teeth can be highly beneficial.

5. Optimally, teeth should be cleaned up about two weeks prior to surgery to reduce the amount of bacteria present in the mouth and lessen the chances of post-operative infection. Laser curettage in the sulcus around each tooth can dramatically reduce the presence of bacteria even further.

6. General medical clearance, especially with older patients should be obtained.

7. A written informed consent signed by the patient should be obtained prior to the planned procedure. All potential complications of the procedure should be thoroughly discussed. It is preferable that a family member also participates in this consent, especially to help verify that all that has been discussed is fully understood. Consideration might be given to a videotaping of the discus-

sion of the consent, which gives the dentist further evidence that all information was discussed and was completely understood by the patient prior to signing the consent form. With the advent of the smartphone, this can be more easily performed than ever before, and the recordings can be readily stored in computer files for easy access in the future.

8. Preoperative medications such as antibiotics should be administered.

9. The oral cavity should be cleansed with an appropriate antimicrobial agent.

10. Local anesthetic **without** a vasoconstrictor should be used. Vasoconstrictors lessen the blood flow in the injected area. Good blood flow to the surgical site is necessary to help assure the best chances of complete healing. Even the transient vasoconstriction produced by anesthetics with a vasoconstrictor can cause enough ischemia to injure the bone and cause local cell death, further impeding rapid and complete healing.

11. Surgery should be performed so that the total lesion can be removed. The surgeon must be skilled in operating around the inferior alveolar nerve (the main nerve that runs through the lower jaw) as well

as operating through the sinus floor and into the sinus. Many times the lesions seen around cavitations, root canal-treated teeth, and untreated CAP teeth are more extensive than they appear on regular X-ray. 3D cone beam imaging of the teeth should always be performed if possible to better plan the surgical approach. It is important to remove all of the diseased tissue. This means that the surgeon should be skilled in operating around all these anatomical structures. Otherwise, the patient should be referred to another surgeon.

12. Usually, the extraction of an infected tooth requires adequate exposure of the bone surrounding the tooth for good visualization in order to access the infected areas. This is obtained by laying a "flap," which simply means that the gum tissue is gently lifted off the bone. The word "gently" is emphasized here since there is a thin layer of tissue that lays directly adjacent to the bone called the periosteum that must be treated with care. The periosteum is the tissue that supplies the outside of the bone with nutrients, and it is also where many of the sensory fibers that can cause post-operative pain are located. It must

be treated with respect and handled gently. The kinder you treat the tissue during any operation the less postoperative complications will occur, and the better healing will proceed.

13. Surgical sites should be irrigated with saline solution or antibiotic solutions that would be acceptable for use in orthopedic surgery. It must be remembered that bone is the tissue being subjected to surgery. Plain water should never be used and medications that have not been evaluated for use in bone elsewhere in the body should also never be used for surgical sites in the jawbone.

14. Extractions should be performed as atraumatically as possible. That means that teeth with more than one root such as molars should usually be sectioned and each root removed individually. This technique avoids fractures of the bone and is kinder to the tissues. Dentists were taught in dental school to "expand the socket" by rocking teeth back and force. The term should be "crack the socket" because cortical bone does not stretch and any expansion is obtained by breaking the surrounding bone. This should be avoided. Surgical removal of bone when indicated is a much better

option and should only be performed with a surgical handpiece (NEVER a dental drill), accompanied by copious sterile saline irrigation (not plain water). Dental drills can introduce air into the surgical site that can form an air embolism. An air embolism is a dangerous situation that can cause death. In addition, dental drills use plain water as an irrigant. This water is not sterile and is not physiologic in terms of salinity. Plain water can cause bone cells to die.

The remainer of the protocol addresses both the proper cleaning of the extracted infected teeth as well as to the cleaning of a cavitation.

15. The approach to cavitation surgery is basically the same as the process followed to clean out the socket where an infected tooth was extracted. After tooth extraction, access to the diseased granulation tissue and bone at the bottom of the tooth socket can be readily obtained. Access to a cavitation site is gained by making a mid-crestal incision and reflection of a full thickness mucoperiosteal flap to the buccal side of the jawbone and extending to the

mucogingival fold. Using a round burr in a surgical handpiece and with copious saline irrigation, an opening is made in the crestal bone large enough to allow complete access to the cavitation.

16. Removal of the infected and ischemic bone can be performed initially with a surgical drill at low revolutions per minute with copious irrigation. It is important to keep the temperature of the bone as cool as possible. Aggressive use of a surgical drill will cause an increase in bone temperature due to friction. The bone cells in contact with the drill will die. The intent of the procedure is to remove dead bone cells and not to produce more dead cells in the process. Most of the surgical debridement should be performed by hand with surgical curettes.

17. The surgical site must be continuously flushed with an irrigation solution such as 0.9% saline solution.

18. Sometimes bone grafting or sinus closure must be performed. Be sure to discuss this with a experienced surgeon.

19. Closure of the surgical site should be accomplished with sutures.

20. Antibiotics should be given postoperatively to prevent re-infection or systemic dissemination of existing infection.
21. Sutures should be removed in seven to ten days.
22. Patients should be instructed to keep pressure on the surgical site by gently biting on surgical gauze. This helps to control bleeding as well as to keep the flap close to the bone during the initial healing phase.
23. Ice should be applied to the side of the face for twenty minutes, then removed for twenty minutes. This should be repeated throughout the entire day of surgery but should not be used the following days.
24. The day after surgery the patient should gently rinse with a mild, warm salt water solution (1/4 teaspoon of salt in an 8 oz. glass of water). This should be done three to four times per day.

Cultures for aerobic and anaerobic bacteria as well as for fungus should be obtained immediately after extraction or entry into a cavitation site to get a "clean catch" sample. A clean catch sample is a sample that consists of only tissue within the surgical site without contamination. By ensuring good isolation and surgical suction, the surgical site will be free from external contamination and the sample will only contain pathogens present within the surgical site, and it will not contain pathogens that may be introduced from the rest of the mouth.

These microbiological samples must be placed in the appropriate culture tubes and the laboratory instructed to let them incubate for at least two weeks. Some of the anaerobic bacteria and fungus take a long time to grow and discarding the sample after just a few days may miss the presence of important pathogens.

Bone tissue samples should be taken from all areas of the surgical site and sent for microscopic analysis by an oral pathologist. Acute and chronic osteomyelitis, osteonecrosis, and other disorders can be determined by microscopic evaluation. The results of the microbiological cultures and tissue pathology will assist in determining the need for any further treatment such as appropriate oral or IV antibiotics.

A Guide to the Optimal Administration of Vitamin C

The causal relationship between vitamin C deficiency and osteoporosis is clear. And in truth, vitamin C deficiencies have been implicated in the causation and/or worsening of most, if not all, chronic degenerative diseases. This is because any area low on vitamin C has increased oxidative stress.

Realizing that an individual with a chronic degenerative disease such as osteoporosis is substantially deficient in vitamin C and the other important components of the general antioxidant matrix in the body is straightforward. However, restoring the levels of vitamin C and other important antioxidants to normal or near-normal levels is not is as simple as one would hope. While popping a vitamin C pill of any size daily will help just about everyone, it falls far short of the goal of reaching the state of optimized health that a normal antioxidant balance will bring in the body.

Many conditions, especially acute infections and acute toxin exposures, can readily be addressed and resolved with an aggressive administration of multigram doses of vitamin C for several days.[1] However, optimizing vitamin C levels in the tissues of the body to minimize the impact and evolution of chronic diseases is a different story. This appendix will endeavor to outline the different ways in which vitamin C can be most effectively administered, along with important suggestions for both reaching and maintaining optimal tissue levels of vitamin C.

Important Factors in the Effective Administration of Vitamin C

1. Dose
2. Route
3. Rate
4. Frequency
5. Duration of treatment period
6. Type of vitamin C
7. Adjunct therapies
8. Safety
9. Quality of overall protocol

1. Dose: The Most Critical Factor for Effective Results

While all of the factors of vitamin C administration to be discussed are important, inadequate dosing is the single most important factor in preventing complete clinical success with the vitamin C treatment. If enough vitamin C is not given to deal with the amount of increased oxidative stress involved with an infection, poisoning, or with an ongoing medical condition, complete clinical success will never be realized. It is also important to emphasize that some success short of an optimal response will always be seen no matter how little vitamin C is given. In sick individuals vitamin C is always in short supply, and any amount will help some. More will help even more. Optimal success will be seen when all excess oxidative stress has been neutralized and continues to be neutralized as it recurs.

In the treatment of acute infections and acute poisonings optimal dosing is especially critical, since many such conditions can be fatal, or they can cause long-term secondary organ damage if present in the body long enough before effective treatment. Determining the initial dose requires clinical evaluation. And even more importantly, follow-up clinical

General Vitamin C Dosage Guide

Vitamin C Type	Typical Dose	Maximum Dose	Dose Frequency	Dose Monitoring/ Adjustments
Liposome-Encapsulated	1,000 to 5,000 mg daily	No absolute dosage	Not necessary to divide into multiple doses	Increase until no further symptomatic improvement
Ascorbyl Palmitate (fat-soluble)	1,000 to 2,000 mg daily	2,000 to 5,000 mg	Best to divide doses throughout day	Increase until no no further symptomatic improvement
Sodium Ascorbate as powder	5 to 15 grams	To bowel tolerance	Best to divide doses throughout day	Bowel tolerance and/or until no further symptomatic improvement

evaluation is needed after the initial dose has been given to determine whether future dosing needs to be higher, the same, or even a little lower. It is always optimal to work with a healthcare practitioner familiar with vitamin C to monitor clinical progress and make dosing changes as indicated.

While not an absolute rule, a reasonable guide for selecting the initial dose of vitamin C to be given intravenously would be roughly from 1 to 1.5 grams per kilogram of body weight. Practically speaking this would mean 25 grams for most children old enough to readily tolerate an IV line, 50 to 75 grams for a 100- to 150-pound person, and 75 to 150 grams for a 150- to 250-pound person. Larger children will benefit most by starting at 50 grams. Lower doses and higher doses can always be given as deemed clinically appropriate.

When determining long-term vitamin C dosing for general healthcare maintenance as well as chronic disease management, factors of convenience, symptom relief, and laboratory test results play significant roles in selecting both the type(s) and amounts of vitamin C to be taken orally daily. The General Vitamin C Dosage Guide on the previous page provides a basic starting reference.

CONVENIENCE

Vitamin C, in capsule, pill, or powder form is best given several times a day due to its rapid clearance through the kidneys. This is less of a concern with the liposome-encapsulated form of vitamin C, as the intracellular uptake of this form of vitamin C substantially slows its excretion, effectively making it a long-acting form of vitamin C. The optimal dosage of regular vitamin C is best determined over a few days by how much sodium ascorbate or ascorbic acid it takes to reach bowel tolerance (just before the onset of diarrhea). Most reasonably healthy individuals will end up with a bowel tolerance dose throughout the day between 5 and 15 grams of vitamin C. Some people have much more sensitive bowels and cannot take more than one or two grams. Such individuals should take more of the liposome-encapsulated vitamin C, as bowel tolerance is not an issue with that form of vitamin C. Other individuals have very high bowel tolerances of 20, 30, 40 grams or more of vitamin C, and a handful of individuals cannot consistently reach a bowel tolerance level. Generally these individuals have significant toxin levels in their bodies, often secondary to dental infections, such as root canal-treated teeth and untreated teeth with chronic apical periodontitis (CAP).

SYMPTOM RELIEF

Very few individuals have completely symptom-free lives. As all symptoms are mediated by increased oxidative stress in some area of the body, at least vitamin C can always be expected to lessen a symptom when dosed correctly. Individuals who begin supplementing vitamin C quickly develop a sense for what amount of vitamin C makes them feel the best, and this is a good way to help determine long-term dosing. Other individuals who have no discernible symptoms will nevertheless begin to develop an increased "health awareness" the longer they supplement vitamin C. Such individuals often begin to feel better without having realized they were not feeling optimally before. Also, they quickly realize when they are having a toxic or infectious challenge, as their sense of wellness becomes slightly impaired. In these instances the vitamin C dose can be increased above maintenance levels for a few days to deal with that challenge and not permit outright sickness to develop.

LABORATORY TESTING

Rarely do all the numbers in a broad array of baseline laboratory tests fall within the reference or normal range. As vitamin C is administered over time many abnormal tests will significantly improve or even normalize. An astute healthcare practitioner will be able to determine optimal doses over time through evaluation of routine laboratory testing. Laboratory testing is an especially elegant way to fine-tune vitamin C dosing, as some individuals may still feel well even while certain laboratory test scores are moving in the wrong direction. An increasing C-reactive protein (CRP) level especially warrants concern.

2. Route: What's the Best Avenue for Vitamin C Administration?

Vitamin C can be given intravenously, intramuscularly, by mouth, per rectum, by misting inhalers, topically on the eyes or in the ears, and both on the skin as well as through it (transdermally). Most commonly it is given orally and intravenously. The success of any vitamin C treatment, however, depends primarily on getting vitamin C molecules in direct contact with the pro-oxidant molecules in the site(s) of increased oxidative stress.

When using vitamin C in the treatment of delicate areas, such as the eyes or the respiratory tract, it is important to always use pH-neutral solutions of vitamin C (sodium ascorbate or properly buffered ascorbic acid). Intramuscular injections, discussed further below, are great for babies and small children. Rectal administrations can also be an option if oral or intravenous routes are not feasible or if a retention enema application is being used, as for a condition such as chronic ulcerative colitis. Conditions such as colitis do not require rectal administration however. Any inflammatory condition of the intestine or colon can also be very effectively treated by oral administration of sodium ascorbate powder in water or juice up to bowel tolerance, or by an intravenous application.

3. Rate: How Fast Should Vitamin C Be Administered?

How fast a dose of vitamin C is given intravenously is a very important factor for maximizing the benefit of vitamin C therapy. Depending on the condition being treated and the effect that is desired, vitamin C can be given in seconds as an IV push or it can be infused rapidly, slowly, or even as a continuous infusion over 24 or more hours.

IV PUSH

When a patient is in imminent danger of death, such as might be seen after an acute exposure to life-threatening amounts of venom or toxin that are still largely circulating in the bloodstream, multigram doses of vitamin C (sodium ascorbate or well-buffered ascorbic acid) can be admnistered via IV push. The idea is to get as much vitamin C in direct contact with circulating toxins as rapidly as possible. The results can be dramatic. Dr. Klenner described how he treated a cyanotic patient who was acutely poisoned by the bite of a venomous Puss Caterpillar only 10 minutes earlier and complaining of severe chest pain, the inability to take a deep breath, and the feeling that he was dying:

> **"Twelve grams of vitamin C was quickly pulled into a 50 c.c. syringe and with a 20 gauge needle was given intravenously as fast as the plunger could be pushed. Even**

**before the injection was completed, he ex-
claimed, 'Thank God.' The poison had been
neutralized that rapidly."**[2]

RAPID INFUSION

Rapid infusion generally means an infusion rate
that is as rapid as a wide-open IV line will permit.
Practically speaking, this translates to 500 to 700 cc
of vitamin C solution being administered in a time
frame between 40 and 60 minutes, typically containing between 50 and 100 grams of vitamin C.

When such an amount of vitamin C is infused
this rapidly the pancreas perceives the vitamin C
load as a glucose load because glucose and vitamin C
molecules are extremely similar chemically.
Consequently the pancreas secretes substantial
insulin into the blood to deal with what it considers
to be an acute excess of glucose. For most individuals the insulin release is significant enough that
a pronounced hypoglycemia, sometimes as low as
20 to 25 mg/dL, ensues and is maintained until the
IV is completed or some oral or IV forms of glucose
are supplied to increase the glucose level. This type
of vitamin C infusion, then, can be viewed as an
endogenously-induced form of insulin potentiation
therapy (IPT).

IPT, involving the deliberate induction of
substantial hypoglycemia with insulin injections,
has been documented to be a very effective way to
increase the cellular uptake of most nutrients and/

or medications given at the same time.[3] IPT is often used to give lower doses of chemotherapy to cancer patients. The endogenously-induced IPT will have the same effect, assuring a much larger uptake of vitamin C into the cells than would otherwise take place when it is infused at a slower rate and no significant release of insulin is stimulated. In cell studies insulin has been documented to stimulate vitamin C uptake and accumulation.[4-6] Such studies, along with known effects of IPT, reliably indicate that similar mechanisms are in play for insulin promoting vitamin C uptake in all the metabolically active cells in the body.

SLOW INFUSION

As noted, rapid infusions can acutely push much more vitamin C inside the cells. However a much greater portion of the vitamin C also ends up being excreted through the kidneys in the process. Many chronic degenerative disease patients, including heart patients and cancer patients, will benefit optimally when their infusions take place over two or more hours. Many such patients will benefit from both rapid and slow infusions during the course of their protocol administration. Vitamin C, like regular antibiotic therapy, can offer more benefit when given several times as a high-concentration, rapidly-infused "loading dose," to be followed over a more extended period of time with repeated slow infusions. This simply allows the underlying disease to be exposed to more vitamin C more of the time, often resulting in dramatic symptom lessening and even disease reversal.

CONTINUOUS INFUSION

This is a form of administration that should be of great value but has not yet been done with any frequency. Dr. Klenner first made the suggestion with regard to the possible treatment of cancer:

> **"This is the reason we believe a dose range of 100 grams to 300 grams daily by continuous intravenous drip for a period of several months might prove surprisingly profitable."** [7]

Perhaps the only flaw in Dr. Klenner's assertion is that it would seem unlikely that most cancers would require months to resolve with such an approach. Of course the practical "flaw" is that as of the writing of this book virtually no hospitals in the United States will permit any infusion of vitamin C, much less a continuous infusion. Should circumstances ever permit this approach, however, it is likely that an enormous amount of good could be done not only with cancer, but also with any other chronic degenerative disease, including neurological conditions like multiple sclerosis and Alzheimer's disease. A practical point, however, would be to hang fresh IV bags of vitamin C every three to four hours, since significant oxidation would occur if the the total 24-hour dose was in one IV bag.

4. Frequency: What's the Optimal Interval Between Vitamin C Administrations?

The appropriate frequency of vitamin C dosing in any of its forms is completely based on the clinical response to the previous administration(s) of vitamin C. When treating an acute infectious disease or an acute intoxication/poisoning, the improvement of vital signs and the reported relief of any associated acute symptomatology dictate how soon and how sizeable the next dose of vitamin C should be. When no significant improvement is seen more vitamin C should be given immediately and generally infused more rapidly. IV push should be reserved for those circumstances when death or coma appear imminent.

If an appropriately-sized dose of vitamin C is administered the first time a positive response should nearly always result, especially if intravenous administration is being utilized. The decision of when and how much the second dose of vitamin C should be will still be dictated by the clinical expertise of the treating healthcare practitioner. An oral vitamin C regimen can also be pushed in a vigorous fashion by a caregiver at home if no healthcare provider is involved. The lowering of elevated temperatures, rapid heart rates, and rapid breathing, along with normalization of elevated or depressed blood pressures and the overall increased comfort level of the patient are the most important parameters to follow in the early stage of treatment. It is also important to give sizeable doses of both regular vitamin C and liposome-encapsulated vitamin C orally regardless of whether the patient is also receiving any intravenous administrations.

5. Duration: How Long Should Vitamin C Administrations Be Continued?

Especially for significant acute infectious diseases, the duration of a vitamin C treatment regimen by whatever route of administration, is important. A patient can and usually does respond very dramatically to a large initial dose of vitamin C. However, even when clinical normalcy appears to have been restored it is very important to give sizeable doses of vitamin C for at least 48 hours after the patient "appears" completely cured. Many infections, especially viral ones, can rebound promptly when vitamin C therapy is not extended for this additional length of time. Giving a large amount of vitamin C orally, IV, and/or IM every 4 to 6 hours around the clock will reliably resolve an acute infectious syndrome much more rapidly than would be seen with a very large single dose with no follow-up dose for another 24 hours.

Vitamin C Type	Advantages	Disadvantages
Liposome-Encapsulated	• Highest bioavailability • No digestive upset or diarrhea • Slower excretion rate • Best intracellular delivery	• Most expensive
CAUTION: *Inexpensive brands are often just emulsions and not truly liposome-encapsulated.*		
Ascorbic Acid	• Most desirable regular form if no concern of stomach upset • Inexpensive	• Frequent dosing and potential of diarrhea can make less convenient • Most prone to stomach upset
Sodium Ascorbate	• Best tolerated of pill/powder forms if large doses are desired • Sodium content not a concern for those worried about fluid retention or high blood pressure • Inexpensive	• Frequent dosing and potential of diarrhea can make less convenient
Calcium Ascorbate	• Calcium acts as buffer, easier on stomach	• More expensive than other forms
CAUTION: *Added calcium is always undesirable.*		
Magnesium Ascorbate	• Brings magnesium and ascorbate into body	• More expensive than other forms
Potassium Ascorbate	• Brings potassium into the body	• More expensive than other forms • Limited to small doses • Requires a measure of regular monitoring
CAUTION: *Potassium can be toxic — too much can be fatal.*		
Other Forms of Ascorbate	• Brings other trace elements into the body	• More expensive than other common forms • Limited to small doses
CAUTION: *Not recommended.* Potential of toxicity if dosed excessively		
Ascorbyl Palmitate	• Fat-soluble, so it provides extra protection for fat-rich tissues • Less potential for digestive upset	• More expensive than other forms

6. Type: What's the Best Chemical Form of Vitamin C to Use?

The essence of vitamin C is its ascorbate anion. The associated cations include the following:

✓ Hydrogen (ascorbic acid)
✓ Sodium (ascorbate)
✓ Calcium (ascorbate)
✓ Magnesium (ascorbate)
✓ Potassium (ascorbate)
✓ Manganese (ascorbate)
✓ Zinc (ascorbate)
✓ Molybdenum (ascorbate)
✓ Chromium (ascorbate)

ASCORBIC ACID

This is really the prototypical form of vitamin C. This is always a desirable form of vitamin C to take when there is no concern with stomach upset due to excess acid effect, or no concern of excess acidity causing pain at the catheter site when given intravenously after being appropriately buffered.

SODIUM ASCORBATE

This is probably the optimal form of regular vitamin C that has not been encapsulated with liposomes. This is because very large amounts can be given up to the point of inducing a diarrhea-like, vitamin C-flush effect when what is known as bowel

tolerance is reached. If exceeding the bowel tolerance level is well-tolerated this is also a very desirable effect as it neutralizes and eliminates a large
amount of gut-generated toxins before they get
absorbed. The amount of sodium ascorbate needed
to exceed the bowel tolerance point can also be
useful as a rough guide to the degree of infection
or toxicity that is present in the patient. Generally,
the greater the infectious and/or toxic challenge the
more vitamin C gets absorbed from the gut and the
less of it reaches the colon, with the bowel tolerance
point not being reached as readily. [8,9]

It should also be noted that large amounts
of sodium ascorbate can be taken by most individuals, including those with high blood pressure
and heart disease, without causing fluid retention
or an increase in blood pressure. This is because
it is sodium chloride, not sodium associated with
another anion like ascorbate, citrate, or bicarbonate,
that reliably causes fluid retention and aggravates
high blood pressure in individuals sensitive to
volume overload. The term "sodium-dependent"
hypertension should forever be replaced with the
term "sodium chloride-dependent" or "table salt-de-
pendent" hypertension. [10,11] In any event, large doses
of sodium ascorbate should not be avoided for fear
of provoking elevated blood pressure.

CALCIUM ASCORBATE

This form is typically marketed as Ester C or buffered vitamin C. This form just adds another unnecessary source of calcium to the supplementing individual. While it is true that it is easy on the stomach, sodium ascorbate is tolerated just as easily and does not aggravate the preexisting state of calcium excess already present in most older individuals.

MAGNESIUM ASCORBATE

This is an excellent form of vitamin C since it brings both magnesium and ascorbate into the body. The only practical limit to dosage with this form of vitamin C would be the amount that starts to approach bowel tolerance and that results in diarrhea. Probably the main reason against supplementing magnesium ascorbate on a regular basis is that it adds significant cost to what are two exceptionally inexpensive supplements when taken separately.

POTASSIUM ASCORBATE

This is also a good form of ascorbate for supplementation. The only problem is that it is relatively easy to overdose on potassium, which can cause fatal cardiac arrhythmias, especially if it is taken with the same abandon as so many other completely nontoxic supplements. Potassium should never really be taken on a regular basis unless advised or prescribed by a healthcare practitioner who has done appropriate clinical and laboratory testing beforehand. For people who are in need of potassium supplementation this can be a excellent supplement. It just needs some measure of regular monitoring.

THE OTHER FORMS OF ASCORBATE

These are forms other than the specific forms mentioned above. They are not really good forms of vitamin C to ingest in large amounts on a regular basis. While ascorbate has no real toxicity concerns, most of the mineral ascorbates, especially manganese, molybdenum, zinc, and chromium, can very easily be overdone. Also, as mentioned above they are needlessly expensive and do not end up providing the amounts of vitamin C that most individuals should be taking on a regular basis. Better to take a quality supplement with a wide range of minerals along with multigram amounts of sodium ascorbate separately.

ASCORBYL PALMITATE

Unlike all the other ascorbate forms listed above, this is a form of vitamin C that is fat-soluble. Including at least a gram or two of ascorbyl palmitate in a daily supplementation regimen can provide important additional antioxidant coverage in fat-rich tissues and areas not otherwise well-protected by the more common forms of vitamin C.[12-14] Ascorbyl palmitate has been demonstrated to protect the cell membrane of intact red blood cells[15] as well as to protect important anti-atherosclerotic lipoproteins in the body.[16] It has also been employed as an antioxidant to prevent skin aging.[17] Liposome delivery systems containing ascorbyl palmitate have been demonstrated to kill cancer cells *in vitro* as well as to slow tumor growth in mice more effectively than with free ascorbic acid.[18] All of these studies indicate the importance of including ascorbyl palmitate as part of an optimally effective vitamin C-centered protocol.

"VITAMIN C COMPLEX"

There is also a vitamin C supplement being marketed as "Vitamin C Complex," with the basic assertion that vitamin C must be present in a "food form" with multiple associated substances, such as antioxidant bioflavonoids like rutin and quercetin, to be of any benefit. Many of the sellers of a product like this even make the incredibly outlandish assertion that pure vitamin C, as ascorbic acid or sodium ascorbate, is not of much benefit and will not even reverse scurvy by itself. In a nutshell, this is all marketing hyperbole by companies trying to carve out a piece of the vitamin C sales pie.

Just as has been asserted several times in this book, vitamin C does function optimally with as large a network of other antioxidants as can be assimilated. However, it is completely wrong and frankly ridiculous to assert that it will not reverse scurvy by itself or that it is of very limited utility by itself. All the work of vitamin C pioneer, Frederick Klenner, M.D., with infectious diseases and toxins demonstrated unequivocally the incredible and typically curative value of vitamin C utilized **_by itself_** in high doses in these conditions.[19]

Just as crazy, some sellers of this product claim ascorbic acid is not vitamin C, which is as crazy as a statement can be. Presumably this assertion is made in order to convince vitamin Consumers that their product is the only one that can deliver the many benefits of vitamin C ingestion. Not surprisingly, this form of vitamin C supplementation is substantially more expensive that regular supplemental forms of vitamin C. Although this is a product that will certainly provide benefits, more benefit is available for less money spent on just ascorbic acid or sodium ascorbate. Buyer beware!

7. Adjunct Therapies: Will Vitamin C Administration Compete with Other Treatments?

Unless another therapy is inherently pro-oxidant or toxic in nature, vitamin C will only **_add_** to the desired effects. For example, if an individual is receiving chemotherapy for cancer the vitamin C can neutralize the chemotherapy drug itself if both are circulating in the blood at the same time. The chemotherapy is a toxic, electron-seeking agent, and the vitamin C is an antioxidant, electron-donating agent. When any chemotherapy agent has received the electrons it is seeking it ceases to be toxic and can no longer kill or help to kill a cancer cell. However this effect is easily avoided by staggering the dosing of any inherently toxic drug and any administered vitamin C by a few hours or so. It should also be noted that when vitamin C is given after a cancer chemotherapy agent it helps both to kill the cancer cell even more effectively while also repairing the damage that was done to normal cells by the chemotherapy. When the vitamin C is given before such chemotherapy a greater cancer-killing effect is also seen and many normal cells that would have been damaged are protected by the greater concentration of vitamin C present.

It is also important to note that vitamin C does not interfere with the antimicrobial effects of antibiotics. Quite the contrary, vitamin C enhances the effects of many antibiotics and one should never avoid indicated antibiotic therapy if there is the possibility to take it along with the vitamin C. Vitamin C has many different supportive effects on the immune system [20] including increasing the degree of antibody response to a pathogen. Even though vitamin C can often do the job on a bacterial infection by itself there is no reason to avoid its synergistic effect with an appropriate antibiotic in resolving the infection.

8. Safety: How Safe is Vitamin C?

An important factor in the administration of any therapy to treat a medical condition is how safe it is. Many traditional medical therapies can often have a desired clinical effect, but they can also have a significant side effect or toxicity much of the time. "First, do no harm" continues to be the appropriate standard by which any therapeutic intervention is measured regardless of how effective it might be some of the time.

Except in patients with significant chronic renal insufficiency or chronic renal failure, vitamin C has no definable toxicity. Of course, nearly all drugs have to be administered with caution in patients with kidney failure, and vitamin C is no exception. It should also be noted that many patients with deteriorating kidney function can benefit greatly from well-monitored vitamin C therapy. This is because inflammation, which is only another way of describing increased oxidative stress, is at the root of evolving kidney failure, like all other chronic degenerative diseases.

Outside of the context of poor kidney function vitamin C is enormously safe given in the highest of doses over extended periods of time in even the sickest of patients.[21] Also, vitamin C has no relation to the development of kidney stones in spite of the continued efforts by the scientific media to convince doctors and the public otherwise. In fact vitamin C reliably decreases the chances of kidney stones and the persons with the highest blood levels of vitamin C have the lowest incidence of kidney stone disease.

One very rare side effect of vitamin C can occur in patients with G6PD deficiency, an X-linked recessive hereditary disease. G6PD (glucose-6-phosphate dehydrogenase) is an enzyme that is especially important in red blood cell metabolism. When is it severely deficient in the red blood cells, a hemolysis (rupture) of many of the red blood cells can be provoked by any of a number of agents, anemia and darkened urine being the result of an acute hemolysis.

The blood test measuring G6PD is readily available, and it is appropriate to obtain this test before initiating vitamin C therapy if possible. However, even when this deficiency is present it is still unlikely that the vitamin C will provoke any red blood cell hemolysis.

If a test is positive and the need for vitamin C is urgent, treatment should proceed, but with closer clinical monitoring, slower infusion, lower doses, and a slower increasing of the vitamin C dose over time. It should also be noted that the initial doses of vitamin C can gradually decrease the susceptibility of the red blood cells to subsequent hemolysis, since vitamin C helps to bolster intracellular glutathione levels, which strongly protects them from hemolysis.

When time permits, the administration of other agents that increase intracellular glutathione levels inside the red blood cells (N-acetyl cysteine, whey protein, liposome-encapsulated glutathione) can also stabilize the red blood cells and increase their resistance to hemolysis before the initiation of vitamin C therapy.

9. Overall Protocol of Administration

This factor is much more important in the treatment of chronic degenerative diseases than when treating acute infectious diseases or acute toxin exposures. Toxins and infections will generally respond favorably and rapidly to the aggressive administration of vitamin C as discussed above. However, how effective it is with a chronic condition depends on how effectively several other factors that use up the antioxidant capacity of the body are addressed. These factors are:

- ✓ How effectively new toxins are being avoided
- ✓ How completely chronic infections and occult acute infections have been eradicated
- ✓ How effectively old toxins have been eliminated and how effectively they are continuing to be eliminated in the most minimally toxic manner possible
- ✓ Whether deficient levels of critical regulatory hormones (testosterone,

estrogen, and thyroid) have been
restored to normal
✓ Whether appropriate prescription
   medications have been utilized

Multi-C Protocol

As the ultimate goal of an optimally effective vitamin C protocol is to get as much of the active (reduced) vitamin C into as many areas of the body in the highest concentrations possible, the Multi-C Protocol utilizes multiple forms of vitamin C for supplementation. The basic outline of this protocol is as follows:

1. One to five grams of liposome-encapsulated vitamin C taken orally daily.
2. Multigram doses of sodium ascorbate powder taken orally several times daily in juice or water up to or reaching bowel tolerance (the induction of watery diarrhea).
3. One to three grams daily of ascorbyl palmitate orally daily.
4. 25 to 150 grams of vitamin C intravenously up to several times weekly and occasionally daily depending on the condition and the need to get vitamin C blood levels at very high levels for longer periods of time.

The reasoning behind the Multi-C Protocol is as follows:

When choosing a
liposome-encapsulated vitamin C...

An additional practical point is that it is very important to take a supplement with a high concentration of liposomes of an appropriately tiny size. Although advertised otherwise, many commercial formulations, as well as homemade formulations, are emulsions only and have zero liposome content.

An emulsion can contain two or more substances that do not normally go into solution, like fat and water, in what can be characterized as a smooth watery suspension containing small fat globules. However, these globules are as much larger than liposomes as a house is larger than a grain of sand. There are none of the unique intracellular biodelivery characteristics of incredibly tiny liposomes shared by large globules of fat. And these globules do not contain vitamin C, anyway.

An emulsified supplement containing vitamin C and lecithin-derived phosphatidylcholine can certainly provide some clinical benefit since both substances are individually quality supplements. Phosphatidylcholine has been demonstrated to have multiple positive effects. [27-31] However, an emulsion does not have the ability to put anything directly inside cells without the consumption of energy like liposomes of the appropriately tiny size.

Once again, buyer beware, as multiple manufacturers are trying to jump on the liposome bandwagon without going through the substantial expense and care involved in producing a consistently high-quality product. The benefits of vitamin C properly encapsulated in liposomes are literally exponentially better that the same amount of vitamin C delivered orally in an emulsion just containing phosphatidylcholine.

1. Liposome-Encapsulated Vitamin C

Liposomes utilize a very unique biodelivery system, achieving an intracellular delivery of a substantial percentage of their payload[22,23] without the expenditure of energy in the process. When that payload is vitamin C the result is cells containing more vitamin C leading to decreased intracellular oxidative stress without an accompanying depletion of the energy resources in the body in order to achieve that goal.

All other forms of regular unencapsulated vitamin C, administered either orally or intravenously, need to consume energy for cells to end up with an increased content of active reduced vitamin C. While oxidized vitamin C circulating in the blood can be taken into cells passively without the immediate consumption of energy, energy must still be spent inside the cells to reduce it back to its active antioxidant state.[24,25]

Reduced (unoxidized) vitamin C circulating in the blood, however, requires an active transport mechanism to get inside the cell, which means that energy must be consumed for the transport system to work.[26] Therefore, even when regular vitamin C is delivered straight into the blood, significant energy consumption must take place to increase the levels of active vitamin C inside the cells.

Liposome-encapsulated vitamin C, even though taken orally, does not deplete any of the energy stores in the body to deliver its payload inside the cells.

In addition to their energy-sparing system of delivery, liposomes have an exceptionally rapid and enhanced form of absorption in the gastrointestinal tract. Unlike regular forms of vitamin C, nearly all of the liposome-encapsulated vitamin C is absorbed.[27]

The payload encapsulation by lipids also prevents potential stomach upset by the liposome contents (in this case, vitamin C). It also prevents any premature breakdown or degradation of the liposome contents that might otherwise occur from enzyme and/or stomach acid exposure.

In the case of liposome-encapsulated vitamin C, there is no issue of bowel tolerance and diarrhea as is seen with regular forms of vitamin C, although a very large dose of liposomes could potentially result in oily, greasy stools in a few individuals.

For all these reasons the unique intracellular delivery of vitamin C encapsulated in liposomes makes it an essential part of any protocol that strives to optimize support of intracellular vitamin C and antioxidant levels.

2. Sodium Ascorbate Powder

The consumption of vitamin C on a regular (optimally daily) basis as sodium ascorbate powder facilitates the direct neutralization of toxins that are formed by the incomplete digestion, or putrefaction, of different foods. When the doses are pushed high enough and bowel tolerance is reached, further intake results in a watery diarrhea. This watery diarrhea, also known as a C-flush, further ensures that a substantial amount of toxins are directly eliminated without the need for neutralization. Inducing a C-flush at least once weekly is a great idea for general health support, as it allows for toxins to be eliminated, toxins to be neutralized, and it helps keep the bowels regular even when the amounts of vitamin C being ingested are not up to bowel tolerance levels. If desired, inducing a C-flush even more frequently is fine.

Anything that induces at least one bowel movement per day, and preferably twice a day, will definitely promote good health. When ingested foodstuffs stay in the gut for more than 24 hours, significant putrefaction and anaerobic bacterial toxin formation will always result. Because of this, any degree of constipation is a substantial additional challenge to maintaining a healthy level of vitamin C and other antioxidants in the body, as many of the most potent toxins generated in a sluggish gut are equal in toxicity to those seen in chronic dental infections, like root canals and other chronically (or acutely) infected teeth, like untreated teeth with CAP.

The regular ingestion of sodium ascorbate also assures a regular uptake of vitamin C into the extracellular fluids and spaces of the body. Just as the liposome-encapsulated vitamin C targets the intracellular spaces the vitamin C powder continually supplies the extracellular areas while providing all of its other benefits in producing a healthy gut. Of course, some of the extracellular vitamin C also eventually makes its way inside the cells as well, just not with the efficiency of oral liposome-encapsulated vitamin C.

3. Ascorbyl Palmitate

As discussed in greater detail above, ascorbyl palmitate is a unique form of vitamin C that is fat-soluble rather than water-soluble. As such, this allows the antioxidant effects of vitamin C to reach areas normally not as readily accessible to regular water-soluble vitamin C.

4) Intravenous Vitamin C (IVC)

IVC allows the administration of vastly higher doses of vitamin C than can be given by any other route. It results in very high concentrations in the blood and extracellular fluids. It also eventually increases intracellular vitamin C levels as well, even though energy consumption is required to achieve this (see above). Although all forms of vitamin C have been documented to have potent antitoxic and antimicrobial properties, a very large body of scientific evidence collected since the early 1940's has shown that properly dosed and administered IVC can result in a degree of toxin (poison) neutralization and infection resolution that simply has not been rivaled by any other agent.[32]

It is also important to emphasize that vitamin C need not be used *instead* of other traditional agents for combating toxins and infections, as it works well *along with* any other traditional measures used for these conditions. However, the evidence does clearly show that vitamin C works better as a monotherapy than any other single agent that modern medicine has to offer.

Another parenteral (non-oral) application of vitamin C that is little used today but that can be highly effective in certain situations is the intramuscular route. Frederick Klenner, MD, who singularly pioneered the field of the effective clinical applications of vitamin C, would often use intramuscular injections in young patients who were not optimal candidates for taking anything intravenously or for ingesting sufficient quantities of anything orally. Regarding the intramuscular injection of vitamin C, Dr. Klenner had the following to say:

> "In small patients, where veins are at a premium, ascorbic acid can easily be given intramuscularly in amounts up to two grams at one site. Several areas can be used with each dose given. Ice held to the gluteal muscles until red, almost eliminates the pain. We always reapply the ice for a few minutes after the injection. Ascorbic acid is also given, by mouth, as followup treatment. Every emergency room should be stocked with vitamin C ampoules of sufficient strength so that time will never be counted—as a factor in saving a life. The 4 gram, 20 c.c. ampoule and 10 gram 50 c.c. ampoule must be made available to the physician." [33]

It should also be noted that the typical injection used by Dr. Klenner was sodium ascorbate or ascorbic acid buffered with sodium bicarbonate, not just straight ascorbic acid. Additionally, great care needs to be taken to ensure that the entire injection is intramuscular, with none of it in the loose subcutaneous tissue. Whether by misguided intramuscular injection or by an infiltrated intravenous infusion of vitamin C, subcutaneous placement of any amount of vitamin C is enormously painful, often for up to an hour or so before resolving. While no damage is done by a subcutaneous infiltration, the pain is significant enough that the patient might not be so willing to permit future vitamin C infusions or injections.

A suggested formula for intramuscular injections would be:

- ✓ 2 cc of vitamin C (500 mg/cc)
- ✓ 1 cc of sterile water,
- ✓ 0.5 cc of 8.4% sodium bicarbonate
- ✓ 1 cc of 2% procaine

(*Formula courtesy of Jason West, DC, NMD*)

This makes a total volume of 4.5 cc, half injected into each buttock.

While Dr. Klenner gave 2 grams rather than 1 gram at each injection site, this protocol eliminates any significant pain resulting from these injections.

Practical IVC Considerations

In addition to how quickly vitamin C should be infused and how much should be given at a time, as discussed above, it is very important that the patient is completely comfortable and free of discomfort or pain in the process. Significant pain during the infusion of vitamin C, or anything else for that matter, will reliably lead to phlebitis, or inflammation of the vein, if not promptly addressed at the time of the infusion. No matter how good a vitamin C-centered protocol might be, it will do little or no good if the patient becomes severely noncompliant in returning for continued IV infusions. Since it is clear that most patients will get their best clinical results with optimally-dosed vitamin C versus other traditional therapies, it is important not to let the patient get to the point of refusing further IVC treatment.

It should first be emphasized that most patients have no problem with vitamin C infusions, tolerating them without any symptomatology of any kind. However, when significant discomfort appears during an IV infusion, the following factors should all be considered in making the infusion as comfortable as possible:

1. **Size of intravenous cannula, or infusion catheter.** A larger cannula inside a smaller vein can cause discomfort.
2. **Placement of cannula.** Even though a cannula might be completely inside the vein, demonstrating venous backflow when tested, pain can ensue when the angle of the cannula abuts directly against the side of the vein or when a venous valve is at the tip of the cannula.

Oftentimes nothing will stop the pain except cannula removal with reinsertion at another site in the vein, with greater care to insert the cannula in as vein-centered an alignment as possible.

3. **Size of the vein**. While some individuals can tolerate IV infusions in the tiniest of veins, many cannot. The largest vein available should always be chosen except when it is already known that smaller, more distal veins tolerate the infusion well, as in a larger man with substantially-sized veins on the back of the hand. If the patient is a smaller woman, or even a child, consideration should be given to having a central line placed if there appears to be no other way to get the amount of vitamin C infused at the rate desired and repeated infusions are clearly warranted for the condition.

4. **Rate of flow**. Many individuals tolerate a slower infusion perfectly well, while always noticing increasing discomfort the more rapid the infusion becomes. If this sensitivity is severe, consideration should again be given to the placement of a central line if deemed appropriate. Some patients will complain of discomfort and get relief when the infusion rate is slowed and then later not feel any discomfort when the infusion rate is once again increased. Whatever the physiological reason is, it appears that the vein can show increased tolerance the longer it is exposed to the vitamin C infusion.

Minimal discomfort can often be alleviated with cold (or even hot!) compresses gently applied and held over the infusion site.

5. **Concentration**. When a large enough vein cannot be found for infusion without significant discomfort a more dilute infusion of vitamin C is usually warranted.

6. **Temperature of the infusion solution**. Making sure the infusion solution is close to body temperature during the administration period can prevent a substantial amount of discomfort from ever developing in the first place. Many offices are quite cold and the IV solutions often tend to be room temperature, or less. One or more refrigerated vitamin C vials should be pre-warmed before addition to a room temperature bag. To minimize any degradation (oxidation) of the vitamin C place the IV bag in hot water for 10 to 15 minutes before adding the vitamin C. The vitamin C vial can similarly be warmed immediately before being added to the IV bag.

7. **Presence of other solutes**. Generally, it is best to infuse vitamin C and nothing else. While other agents can be added, it is important not to blame the vitamin C for discomfort in the IV when something else is at fault.

8. **pH of the infusion**. The more acidic an infusion is the more likely it will hurt. A pH of 7.0 to 7.4 is ideal, and it is characteristically reached when sodium ascorbate powder is put into solu-

tion in sterile water. When ascorbic acid is used it must be buffered with sodium bicarbonate. Vials of ascorbic acid buffered with sodium bicarbonate are available but they are generally buffered only to be somewhere in the range of pH 5.5 to 7.0. For the exceptionally sensitive patient, pH test paper should be utilized to make sure pH is in the optimal range and more sodium bicarbonate should be added to the infusion if necessary to get into that range.

9. **Nature of carrier solution**. Generally it is best to infuse vitamin C mixed in sterile water. While D5W, normal saline, or lactated Ringer's solution can be used, it is best to stick with vitamin C in sterile water, buffered as close to a pH of 7.0 to 7.4 as possible. D5W should really never be used, since it puts more glucose into the blood at the same time as the vitamin C and it prevents the maximal amount of vitamin C from getting into the cells, since glucose and vitamin C use the same mechanism for entering the cells.

10. **Presence of persistent or severe pain**. Any extravasation, or leakage, of vitamin C outside of the vein and into the subcutaneous tissue is severely painful, usually persisting for an hour or more before dissipation is complete. Sometimes the cannula can move back out of the vein transiently and a little leakage will take place. When the cannula comes completely

out of the vein it will be obvious to the experienced practitioner.

11. **Vitamin C-induced hypoglycemia**. Rarely, some individuals are so sensitive to the infusion of multigram amounts of vitamin C that they will demonstrate some hypoglycemia secondary to increased insulin release from the pancreas at infusion rates well below what most other patients tolerate easily. When any unexplained agitation, sweating, minimal disorientation, or increase in blood pressure occurs, be prepared to give some fruit juice orally or some glucose intravenously. Also, while very rare, an occasional individual, typically cachetic and poorly nourished in general, can have a delayed hypoglycemia reaction hours later at home. All patients should be encouraged to promptly eat after an infusion session is complete.

12. **Allergy-like reactions**. Technically, the ascorbate anion should never cause an allergic reaction in anyone as it is a natural antioxidant molecule vital to health, as well as a substance that can be used to *treat* an allergic reaction. Nevertheless, individuals may sometimes (rarely) demonstrate a rash and feel poorly. When this occurs shortly after the IV is started a allergy-like reaction is likely and the IV should be stopped. Consideration should then be given to obtaining vitamin C from a different source. Corn is commonly a source, but beet and casaba

are also sources. When the reaction occurs late in the IV or shortly after its conclusion a detoxification from the cells is more likely. This type of reaction and how to deal with it is addressed below in the "Mop-Up Vitamin C" section. If different types of vitamin C, mixed in different carrier solutions, continue to produce the same effect, premedication with an injection of 100 to 250 mg of hydrocortisone will usually blunt or prevent the reaction. This is a one-time dose and further steroids should not be given following the infusion.

13. **No local anesthetics**. While used by some practitioners, I am not in favor of giving any types of anesthetic agents that would prevent the perception of pain in the vein. If pain is reported by the patient and pain relief through anesthesia is obtained, the pain-causing inflammation in the vein can still result in enough of a reaction that vein thrombosis and subsequent sclerosis can occur. Relieving infusion pain with anesthesia is not a good idea for the long-term health of the veins. However, this does not refer to the use of a small amount of lidocaine in the subcutaneous tissue to lessen or block the pain of the initial needle stick for placement of the intravenous cannula if felt indicated.

Mop-Up IVC

Many individuals, especially sicker ones with acute and chronic infections as well as substantial toxin accumulations in their bodies, will feel anywhere from minimally to substantially ill late during an infusion of vitamin C or directly following it. These exacerbations of illness have been called Herxheimer, or Herxheimer-like reactions. The first described Herxheimer reaction occurred when syphilis patients with a high pathogen load took their first injection of penicillin. The kill-off of the pathogens was so extensive that massive amounts of pro-oxidant dead pathogen-related debris was released into the blood as a result. The clinical result was a much sicker patient, at least in the short term, while the body processed and eliminated the toxic debris. Following an infusion of vitamin C these Herxheimer-like reactions can occur because of one or more of the following reasons:

1. **Whenever an acute or chronic infection responds dramatically enough to the anti-microbial effect of vitamin C.** This results in the release of toxic pathogen-related debris into the blood and lymphatics similar to the syphilis example above.

2. **Whenever a legitimate detoxification occurs**. When some individuals with long-standing and substantial accumulations of toxins inside the cells receive a high enough dose of vitamin C quickly enough, toxins are then mobilized out of the cells and flood the blood and lymphatics. Generally, this occurs only when toxin levels are so high that many

of the natural enzymatic chelators and toxin mobilizers are themselves in an oxidized and relatively nonfunctional state. The massive administration then causes a big intracellular rise in vitamin C, the enzymes are repaired by reduction (electron donation) from the vitamin C, and the toxins are released in large quantities. It is very important to realize that detoxification is also retoxification, and many newly mobilized toxins are just as free to be redeposited anew somewhere else in the body as to be excreted via the urine or feces. Detoxification should never be deliberately done vigorously without the ability to sufficiently promote neutralization and excretion of those toxins after they are released from the cells.

3. **Whenever a substantial quantity of cancer cells are rapidly killed via necrosis**: When vitamin C is dosed and administered correctly, many different cancers will begin to resolve, often to the point of complete resolution, as necrosis of cancer cells ensues. When a patient has a relatively large physical mass of cancer cells in their body this type of reaction is more likely to occur than when the collective cancer mass is small. This reaction can be very dramatic in some patients and several days may be needed for the patient to properly process and excrete the pro-oxidant debris. Of

note as well, both cancer cells and most infectious agents have very large concentrations of reactive iron inside and the rupture of cancer cells and pathogens via vitamin C-fed mechanisms can quite abruptly release large amounts of reactive iron into the blood and lymphatics. Iron is highly toxic (pro-oxidant) when concentrated in its unbound, reactive form, and it can take up to two weeks to clear from the blood.

The Mop-Up vitamin C infusion, at first, might seem paradoxical. That is to say, the very same agent (vitamin C) that caused the flood of pro-oxidant debris into the blood and lymphatics is also the very same agent best suited to deal with that. The trick is in the amount of vitamin C infused and the rate at which it is infused.

All three of the types of pro-oxidant reactions noted above share one thing in common. Namely, they needed large amounts of vitamin C given quickly to become manifest. However, at the termination of such an infusion a "Low & Slow" follow-up infusion of vitamin C at 25% or less of the initial amount given, infused over two hours or more, will readily "mop-up" much or all of the pro-oxidant debris released by the larger rapid infusion.

The mop-up infusion does not significantly worsen the pro-oxidant release because of its low concentration and slow rate of infusion. However, it does very effectively neutralize the toxins already released while they are circulating in the blood and lymphatics. While the figures are not precise, this would mean that someone who was feeling well at the outset of a 50-gram infusion of vitamin C but began feeling poorly after the completion of the infusion in about one hour, should then receive about 12.5 grams of vitamin C infused over another two hours.

While most pro-oxidant debris release scenarios occur when stimulated, as with a vitamin C infusion, it also important to appreciate what is going on in a patient with an extended, chronic detoxification process. For example, when an older patient has an exceptionally large amount of stored toxins in the body the stage is set for a chronic release of toxins when enough other things occur. The relatively abrupt initiation of a quality supplement regimen, especially when accompanied or preceded by a removal of ongoing sources of toxin exposure, as from dental infections like root canals, can result in enough of a reactivation of natural detoxification enzymes inside the cells that a chronic detoxification results. As such, the patient can begin to feel poorly a greater percentage of the time the less the antioxidant capacity of the body is supported.

Just as with the acute pro-oxidant debris release scenario, the chronic one is readily dealt with by the same "Low & Slow" vitamin C infusions, with a good clinical response typically realized. However, many chronic detoxifications can take months or sometimes years before the individual truly feels well, so experimentation must take place with finding the best amounts of vitamin C to take orally that will neutralize the pro-oxidant products of detoxification without significantly further stimulating their release from the cells.

Another especially important consideration about the Mop-Up vitamin C infusion is that is allows the healthcare practitioners to push vitamin C doses higher than might have been possible otherwise. As long as a patient feels good by the time they leave the office they will generally come back for more treatment, even if they were a bit symptomatic toward the end of the initial infusion. Mop-Up vitamin C, then, is a tool that allows a large group of patients that could otherwise only tolerate substantially lower doses of vitamin C to push their doses into a range that will produce even more positive clinical outcomes that were not otherwise attainable.

Conclusion

All infections, all toxin exposures, and all chronic degenerative diseases will benefit some and often greatly from properly dosed and administered vitamin C. The different forms of vitamin C and the various ways to give it offer a wide range of treatment possibilities, capable of being appropriately individualized for optimal clinical response. The new concept of Mop-Up vitamin C now allows the vitamin C practitioner to push the therapeutic envelope to previously unattainable levels. Utilized properly, vitamin C-centered protocols have already gone and will continue to go where no protocols have gone before.

Examples of Diagnostic Imaging Technology

The use of modern diagnostic tools can give dentists and physicians greatly enhanced ability to diagnose silent oral infections and monitor progress in their treatment. Several side-by-side comparisons between standard 2D panoramic X-rays and 3D cone beam imaging demonstrate the dramatic difference in clarity provided by the latter.

In this appendix you will also see a case study with before and after thermographic images following remediation of CAP in a few teeth. The difference is not only seen around the oral cavity but also in the breast tissue. Decreasing infection decreases the inflammation-associated heat seen in the lymphatics connecting the affected teeth and the breast tissue.

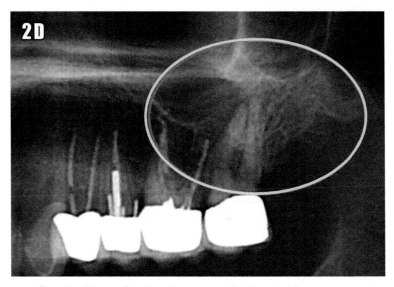

Regular X-ray of tooth with a crown that has not been given endodontic treatment. There is no chronic apical periodontitis (CAP) revealed here.

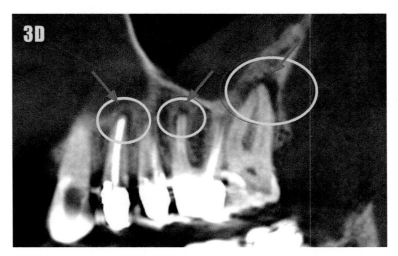

A 3D cone beam image of the tooth shown above reveals a significant CAP defect around that tooth. It also reveals CAP at the roots of two root canal-treated teeth to the left.

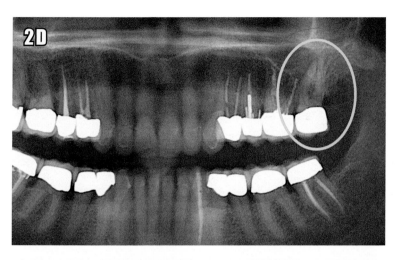

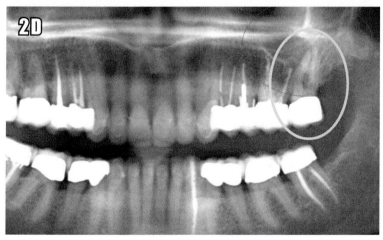

Two different panoramic 2D X-rays show the same
untreated tooth with crown (in yellow circle). No apparent
chronic apical peridontitis (CAP) is seen in either image.
See comparative 3D cone beam images of the same tooth
on the next page.

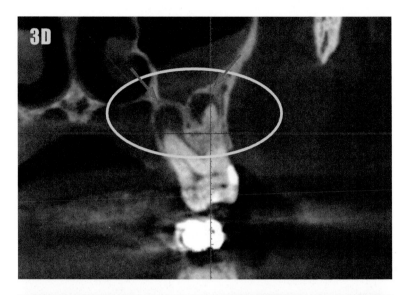

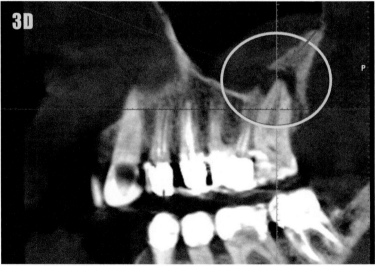

These 3D cone beam images, one from the front and one from the side, reveal large CAP defects with erosion of bone into the maxillary sinus cavity and with an air-fluid level in the sinus.

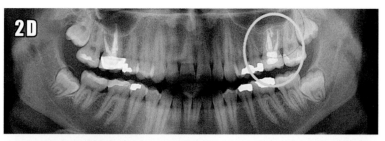

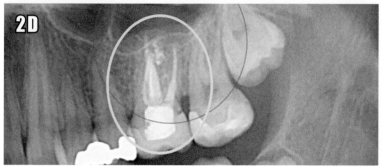

Regular X-rays of this encircled root canal-treated tooth do not reveal any CAP.

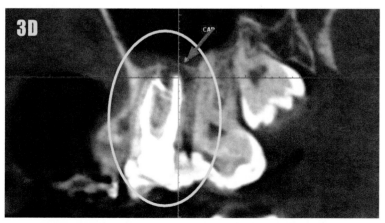

Dark area (radiolucency) around the right root in the 3D image reveals CAP that was undetected in the traditional X-rays shown above.

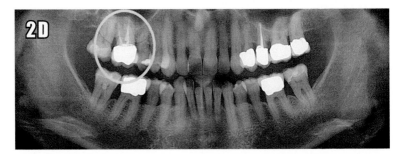

Regular X-ray of encircled root canal-treated tooth shows no
apparent CAP.

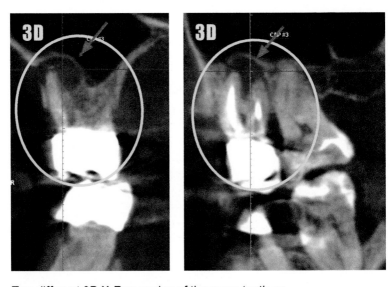

Two different 3D X-Ray angles of the same tooth as
highlighted above show a large CAP defect surrounding
both root tips and with some complete bone erosion allowing
entry into the maxillary sinus above.

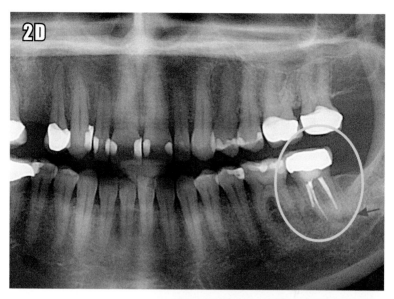

ABOVE: A regular X-ray of a root canal-treated tooth fails to detect any clear CAP defect.

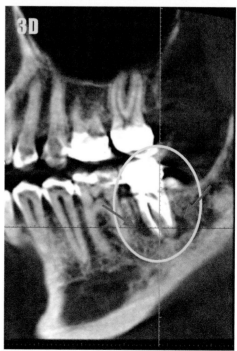

RIGHT: A 3D cone beam image of the same tooth reveals large CAP defects around both roots.

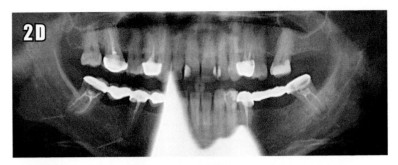

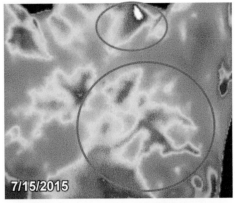

Red arrows on the panoramic X-ray above show three CAP teeth. These and two other teeth were extracted and the gums were treated with ozone.

A thermograph prior to treatment shows a high degree of inflammation-caused heat on the neck and on the left breast as indicated by the white and red areas. Ten months later a thermograph of the same area show a significant reduction in temperatures (inflammation).

These two images suggest a lymphatic connection between infected teeth and other parts of the body, in this case, the neck and breast.

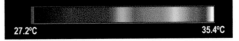

27.2°C   35.4°C

Thermography images courtesy of Three Rivers
Thermography, ThreeRiversThermography.com

References

Chapter 1

1. Kulacz R., Levy T. (2014) *The Toxic Tooth: How a root canal could be making you sick.* Henderson, NV: MedFox Publishing, p. 99-103.

2. Bjorndal L., Reit C. (2004) The annual frequency of root fillings, tooth extractions and pulp-related procedures in Danish adults during 1977-2003. *International Endodontic Journal*, 37:782-788. PMID: 15479261

3. Kamberi B., Hoxha V., Stavileci M. et al. (2011) Prevalence of apical periodontitis and endodontic treatment in a Kosovar adult population. *BMC Oral Health*, 11:32. PMID: 22126237

4. Matijevic J., Cizmekovic Dadic T., Prpic Medicic G. et al. (2011) Prevalence of apical periodontitis and quality root canal fillings in population of Zagreb, Croatia: a cross-sectional study. *Croatian Medical Journal*, 52:679-687. PMID: 22180266

5. Covello F., Franco V., Schiavetti R. et al. (2010) Prevalence of apical periodontitis and quality endodontic treatment in an Italian adult population. *ORAL & Implantology*, 3:9-14. PMID: 23285391

6. Van der Veken D., Curvers F., Fieuwa S., Lambrechts P. (2016) Prevalence of apical periodontitis and root filled teeth in a Belgian subpopulation found on CBCT images. *International Endodontic Journal*, Mar 19 [Epub ahead of print]. PMID: 26992464

7. Ilic J., Vujaskovic M., Tihacek-Sojic L., Milic-Lemic A. (2014) Frequency and quality of root canal fillings in an adult Serbian population. *Srpski Arhiv za Celokupno Lekarstvo*, 142:663-668. PMID: 25730994

8. Jersa I., Kundzina R. (2013) Periapical status and quality of root fillings in a selected adult Riga population. *Stomatologija*, 15:73-77. PMID: 24375309

9. Tsuneishi M., Yamamoto T., Yamanaka R. et al. (2005) Radiographic evaluation of periapical status and prevalence of endodontic treatment in an adult Japanese population. *Oral Surgery, Oral Medicine, Oral Pathology, Oral Radiology, and Endodontics*, 100:631-635. PMID: 16243252

10. Hollanda A., de Alencar A., Estrela C. et al. (2008) Prevalence of endodontically treated teeth in a Brazilian adult population. *Brazilian Dental Journal*, 19:313-317. PMID: 19180320

11. Lopez-Lopez J., Jane-Salas E., Estrugo-Devesa A. et al. (2012) Frequency and distribution of root-filled teeth and apical periodontitis in an adult population of Barcelona, Spain. *International Dental Journal*, 62:40-46. PMID: 22251036

12. Tsuneishi M., Yamamoto T., Yamanaka R. et al. (2005) Radiographic evaluation of periapical status and prevalence of endodontic treatment in an adult Japanese population. *Oral Surgery, Oral Medicine, Oral Pathology, Oral Radiology, and Endodontics*, 100:631-635. PMID: 16243252

13. aae.org http://www.aae.org/about-aae/news-room/endodontic-treatment-statistics.aspx (2017)

14. U.S. Census Bureau, https://www.census.gov/population/www/socdemo/men_women_2006.html (2017)

15. Lemagner F., Maret D., Peters O. et al. (2015) Prevalence of apical bone defects and evaluation of associated factors detected with cone-beam computed tomographic images. *Journal of Endodontics*, 41:1043-1047. PMID: 25917943

16. Segura-Egea J., Castellanos-Cosano L., Machuca G. et al. (2012) Diabetes mellitus, periapical inflammation and endodontic treatment outcome. *Medicina Oral, Patologia Oral y Cirugia Bucal*, 17:e356-e361. PMID: 22143698

17. Rocas I., Siqueira Jr. J., Debelian G. (2011) Analysis of symptomatic and asymptomatic primary root canal infections in adult Norwegian patients. *Journal of Endodontics*, 37:1206-1212. PMID: 21846535

18. Berlinck T., Tinoco J., Carvalho F. et al. (2015) Epidemiological evaluation of apical periodontitis prevalence in an urban Brazilian population. *Brazilian Oral Research*, 29:51. PMID: 25760068

19. Segura-Egea J., Jimenez-Pinzon A., Rios-Santos J. et al. (2008) High prevalence of apical periodontitis amongst smokers in a sample of Spanish adults. *International Endodontic Journal*, 41:310-316. PMID: 18217991

20. Gulsahi K., Gulsahi A., Ungor M., Genc Y. (2008) Frequency of root-filled teeth and prevalence of apical periodontitis in an adult Turkish population. *International Endodontic Journal*, 41:78-85. PMID: 17979966

21. Loftus J., Keating A., McCartan B. (2005) Periapical status and quality of endodontic treatment in an adult Irish population. *International Endodontic Journal*, 38:81-86. PMID: 15667629

22. Jimenez-Pinton A., Segura-Egea J., Poyato-Ferrera M. et al. (2004) Prevalence of apical periodontitis and frequency of root-filled teeth in an adult Spanish population. *International Endodontic Journal*, 37:167-173. PMID: 15009405

23. De Moor R., Hommez G., De Boever J. et al. (2000) Periapical health related to the quality of root canal treatment in a Belgian population. *International Endodontics Journal*, 33:113-120. PMID: 11307451

24. Marques M., Moreira B., Eriksen H. (1998) Prevalence of apical periodontitis and results of endodontic treatment in an adult, Portuguese population. *International Endodontic Journal*, 31:161-165. PMID: 10321161

25. Lupi-Pegurier L., Bertrand M., Muller-Bolla M. et al. (2002) Periapical status, prevalence and quality of endodontic treatment in an adult French population. *International Endodontic Journal*, 35:690-697. PMID: 12196222

26. Chen C., Hasselgren G., Serman N. et al. (2007) Prevalence and quality of endodontic treatment in the Northern Manhattan elderly. *Journal of Endodontics*, 33:230-234. PMID: 17320702

27. De Cleen M., Schuurs A., Wesselink P., Wu M. (1993) Periapical status and prevalence of endodontic treatment in an adult Dutch population. *International Endodontic Journal*, 26:112-119. PMID: 8330933

28. Eckerbom M., Flygare L., Magnusson T. (2007) A 20-year follow-up study of endodontic variables and apical status in a Swedish population. *International Endodontic Journal*, 40:940-948. PMID: 17883402

29. Eriksen H., Bjertness E. (1991) Prevalence of apical periodontitis and results of endodontic treatment in middle-aged adults in Norway. *Endodontics & Dental Traumatology*, 7:1-4. PMID: 1915119

30. Nur B., Ok E., Altunsoy M. et al. (2014) Evaluation of technical quality and periapical health of root-filled teeth by using cone-beam CT. *Journal of Applied Oral Science*, 22:502-508. PMID: 25591019

31. Paes da Silva Ramos Fernandes L., Ordinola-Zapata R., Hungaro Duarte M., Alvares Capelozza A. (2013) Prevalence of apical periodontitis detected in cone beam CT images of a Brazilian subpopulation. *Dento Maxillo Facial Radiology*, 42:80179163. PMID: 22752318

32. Archana D., Gopikrishna V., Gutmann J. et al. (2015) Prevalence of periradicular radiolucencies and its association with the quality of root canal procedures and coronal restorations in an adult urban Indian population. *Journal of Conservative Dentistry*, 18:34-38. PMID: 25657524

33. Asgary S., Shadman B., Ghalamkarpour Z. et al. (2010) Periapical status and quality of root canal fillings and coronal restorations in Iranian population. *Iranian Endodontic Journal*, 5:74-82. PMID: 23130031

34. Huumonen S., Suominen A., Vehkalahti M. (2016) Prevalence of apical periodontitis in root filled teeth: findings from a nationwide survey in Finland. *International Endodontic Journal*, Feb 25 [Epub ahead of print]. PMID: 26919266

35. Oginni A., Adeleke A., Mejabi M., Sotunde O. (2015) Risk factors for apical periodontitis sub-urban adult population. *The Nigerian Postgraduate Medical Journal*, 22:105-109. PMID: 26259158

36. Alfouzan K., Baskaradoss J., Geevarghese A. et al. (2016) Radiographic diagnosis of periapical status and quality of root canal fillings in a Saudi Arabian subpopulation. *Oral Health & Preventive Dentistry*, 14:241-248. PMID: 26669654

37. Mukhaimer R., Hussein E., Orafi I. (2012) Prevalence of apical periodontitis and quality of root canal treatment in an adult Palestinian sub-population. *The Saudi Dental Journal*, 24:149-155. PMID: 23960544

Chapter 2

1. American Institute for Cancer Research, http://www.aicr.org/learn-more-about-cancer/infographics/infographics-economics.html (2017)

2. National Cancer Institute, https://www.cancer.gov/about-cancer/understanding/statistics (2017)

3. Wakizaka A, Aiba N, Okuhara E, Kawazoe Y, Production of 5-formyluracil from thymine in an *in vitro* active oxygen-generating system. *Biochem Int.* 1987 Feb;14(2):289-95. PMID: 3107566.

4. Longjian Liu, Barbara Simon, et al, Impact of diabetes mellitus on risk of cardiovascular disease and all-cause mortality: Evidence on health outcomes and antidiabetic treatment in United States adults, *World J Diabetes.* 2016 Oct 15; 7(18): 449–461. Published online 2016 Oct 15. doi: 10.4239/wjd. v7.i18.449 PMCID: PMC5065665

5. Centers for Disease Control, https://www.cdc.gov/heartdisease/facts.htm (2017)

6. Cardiovascular Disease: A costly burden for America, Projections through 2035, http://www.heart.org/idc/groups/heart-public/@wcm/@adv/documents/downloadable/ucm_491543.pdf, American Heart Association, 2017.

7. American Diabetes Association, http://www.diabetes.org/diabetes-basics/statistics/ (2017)

Chapter 3

1. Gulati M., Anand V., Jain N. et al. (2013) Essentials of periodontal medicine in preventive medicine. *International Journal of Preventive Medicine,* 4:988-994. PMID: 24130938

2. Barilli A., Passos A., Marin-Neto J., Franco L. (2006) Peridontal disease in patients with ischemic coronary atherosclerosis at a University Hospital. *Arquivos Brasileiros de Cardiologia,* 87:695-700. PMID: 17262105

3. Humphrey L., Fu R., Buckley D. et al. (2008) Periodontal disease and coronary artery disease incidence: a systemic review and meta-analysis. *Journal of General Internal Medicine,* 23:2079-2086. PMID: 18807098

4. Dorn J., Genco R., Grossi S. et al. (2010) Periodontal disease and recurrent cardiovascular events in survivors of myocardial infarction (MI): the Western New York Acute MI Study. *Journal of Periodontology,* 81:502-511. PMID: 20367093

5. Ameet M., Avneesh H., Babita R., Pramod P. (2013) The relationship between periodontitis and systemic diseases—hype or hope? *Journal of Clinical and Diagnostic Research,* 7:758-762. PMID: 23730671

6. Hanaoka Y., Soejima H., Yasuda O. et al. (2013) Level of serum antibody against a periodontal pathogen is associated with atherosclerosis and hypertension. *Hypertension Research,*36:829-833. PMID: 23676848

7. Kodovazenitis G., Pitsavos C., Papadimitriou L. et al. (2014) Association between periodontitis and acute myocardial infarction: a case-control study of a nondiabetic population. *Journal of Periodontal Research,* 49:246-252. PMID: 23713486

8. Willershausen I., Weyer V., Peter M. et al. (2014) Association between chronic periodontal and apical inflammation and acute myocardial infarction. *Odontology,* 102:297-302. PMID: 23604464

9. Anitha V., Nair S., Shivakumar V. et al. (2015) Estimation of high sensitivity C-reactive protein in patients with periodontal disease and without coronary artery disease. *Indian Journal of Dental Research,* 26:500-503. PMID: 26672420

10. Bokhari S., Khan A., Leung W., Wajid G. (2015) Association of periodontal and cardiovascular diseases: South-Asian studies 2001-2012. *Journal of Indian Society of Periodontology*, 19:495-500. PMID: 26644713

11. Pessi T., Karhunen V., Karjalainen P. et al. (2013) Bacterial signatures in thrombus aspirates of patients with myocardial infarction. *Circulation*, 127:1219-1228. PMID: 23418311

12. Haraszthy V., Zambon J., Trevisan M. et al. (2000) Identification of periodontal pathogens in atheromatous plaques. *Journal of Periodontology*, 71:1554-1560. PMID: 11063387

13. Mattila K., Pussinen P., Paju S. (2005) Dental infections and cardiovascular diseases: a review. *Journal of Periodontology*, 76:2085-2088. PMID: 16277580

14. Mahendra J., Mahendra L., Kurian V. et al. (2010) 16S rRNA-based detection of oral pathogens in coronary atherosclerotic plaque. *Indian Journal of Dental Research*, 21:248-252. PMID: 20657096

15. Ott S., El Mokhtari N., Rehman A. et al. (2007) Fungal rDNA signatures in coronary atherosclerotic plaques. *Environmental Microbiology*, 9:3035-3045. PMID: 17991032

16. Ott S., El Mokhtari N., Musfeldt M. et al. (2006) Detection of diverse bacterial signatures in atherosclerotic lesions of patients with coronary heart disease. *Circulation*, 113:929-937. PMID: 16490835

17. Ford P., Gemmell E., Chan A. et al. (2006) Inflammation, heat shock proteins and periodontal pathogens in atherosclerosis: an immunohistologic study. *Oral Microbiology and Immunology*, 21:206-211. PMID: 16842503

18. Louhelainen A., Aho J., Tuomisto S. et al. (2014) Oral bacterial DNA findings in pericardial fluid. *Journal of Oral Microbiology*, 6:25835. PMID: 25412607

19. Pyysalo M., Pyysalo L., Pessi T. et al. (2013) The connection between ruptured cerebral aneurysms and odontogenic bacteria. *Journal of Neurology, Neurosurgery, and Psychiatry*, 84:1214-1218. PMID: 23761916

20. Caplan D., Pankow J., Cai J. et al. (2009) The relationship between self-reported history of endodontic therapy and coronary heart disease in the Atherosclerosis Risk in Communities Study. *Journal of the American Dental Association*, 140:1004-1012. PMID: 19654253

21. Joshipura K., Pitiphat W., Hung H. et al. (2006) Pulpal inflammation and incidence of coronary heart disease. *Journal of Endodontics*, 32:99-103. PMID: 16427454

22. Rosenfeld M. (2013) Inflammation and atherosclerosis: direct versus indirect mechanisms. *Current Opinion in Pharmacology*, 13:154-160. PMID: 23357128

23. Legein B., Temmerman L., Biessen E., Lutgens E. (2013) Inflammation and immune system interactions in atherosclerosis. *Cellular and Molecular Life Sciences*, 70:3847-3869. PMID: 23430000

24. Sadighi Shamami M., Sadighi Shamami M., Amini S. (2011) Periodontal disease and tooth loss as risks for cancer: a systematic review of the literature. *Iranian Journal of Cancer Prevention*, 4:189-198. PMID: 26322197

25. Cugini C., Klepac-Ceraj V., Rackaityte E. et al. (2013) *Porphyromonas gingivalis*: keeping the pathos out of the biont. *Journal of Oral Microbiology*, PMID: 23565326

26. Wen B., Tsai C., Lin C. et al. (2014) Cancer risk among gingivitis and periodontitis patients: a nationwide cohort study. *QJM*, 107:283-290. PMID: 24336850

27. Sayehmiri F., Sayehmiri K., Asadollahi K. et al. (2015) The prevalence rate of *Porphyromonas gingivalis* and its association with cancer: a systemic review and meta-analysis. *International Journal of Immunopathology and Pharmacology*, 28:160-167. PMID: 26002887

28. Chung J., Tsai M., Huang C. et al. (2016) A population-based study on the associations between chronic periodontitis and the risk of cancer. *International Journal of Clinical Oncology*, 21:219-223. PMID: 26280747

29. Michaud D., Kelsey K., Papathanasiou E. et al. (2016) Periodontal disease and risk of all cancers among male never smokers: an updated analysis of the Health Professionals Follow-Up Study. *Annals of Oncology*, 27:941-947. PMID: 26811350

30. Shrihari T., Vasudevan V., Manjunath V., Devaraju D. (2016) Potential co-relation between chronic periodontitis and cancer—an emerging concept. *The Gulf Journal of Oncology*, 1:20-24. PMID: 27050175

31. Haladyj A., Kaczynski T., Gorska R. (2016) [The link between periodontitis and pancreatic cancer—review of the literature]. Article in Polish. *Wiadomosci Lekarskie*, 69:87-91. PMID: 27164283

32. Michaud D., Joshipura K., Giovannucci E., Fuchs C. (2007) A prospective study of periodontal disease and pancreatic cancer in US male health professionals. *Journal of the National Cancer Institute*, 99:171-175. PMID: 17228001

33. Chang J., Tsai C., Chen L., Shan Y. (2016) Investigating the association between periodontal disease and risk of pancreatic cancer. *Pancreas*, 45:134-141. PMID: 26474422

34. Hieken T., Chen J., Hoskin T. et al. (2016) The microbiome of aseptically collected human breast tissue in benign and malignant disease. *Scientific Reports*, 6:30751. PMID: 27485780

35. Kostic A., Gevers D., Pedamallu C. et al. (2012) Genomic analysis identifies association of *Fusobacterium* with colorectal carcinoma. *Genome Research*, 22:292-298. PMID: 22009990

36. Castellarin M., Warren R., Freeman J. et al. (2012) *Fusobacterium nucleatum* infection is prevalent in human colorectal carcinoma. *Genome Research*, 22:299-306. PMID: 22009989

37. Idrissi Janati A., Durand R., Karp I. et al. (2016) [Association between oral conditions and colorectal cancer: a literature review and synthesis]. Article in French. *Revue d'Epidemiologie et de Sante Publique*, 64:113-119. PMID: 26923863

38. Rosenquist K. (2005) Risk factors in oral and oropharyngeal squamous cell carcinoma: a population-based case-control study in southern Sweden. *Swedish Dental Journal. Supplement.* 179:1-66. PMID: 16335030

39. Tezal M., Grossi S., Genco R. (2005) Is periodontitis associated with oral neoplasms? *Journal of Periodontology,* 76:406-410. PMID: 15857075

40. Kruger M., Hansen T., Kasaj A., Moergel M. (2013) The correlation between chronic periodontitis and oral cancer. *Case Reports in Dentistry,* 2103:262410. PMID: 23936684

41. Tezal M., Sullivan M., Reid M. et al. (2007) Chronic periodontitis and the risk of tongue cancer. *Archives of Otolaryngology—Head & Neck Surgery,* 133:450-454. PMID: 17515503

42. Inaba H., Sugita H., Kuboniwa M. et al. (2014) *Porphyromonas gingivalis* promotes invasion of oral squamous cell carcinoma through induction of proMMP9 and its activation. Cellular Microbiology, 16:131-145. PMID: 23991831

43. Ha N., Park D., Woo B. et al. (2016) *Porphyromonas gingivalis* increases the invasiveness of oral cancer cells by upregulating IL-8 and MMPs. *Cytokine,* 86:64-72. PMID: 27468958

44. Laprise C., Shahul H., Madathil S. et al. (2016) Periodontal diseases and risk of oral cancer in Southern India: results from the HeNCe Life study. *International Journal of Cancer,* 139:1512-1519. PMID: 27215979

45. Moraes R., Dias F., Figueredo C., Fischer R. (2016) Association between chronic periodontitis and oral/oropharyngeal cancer. *Brazilian Dental Journal,* 27:261-266. PMID: 27224557

46. Gondivkar S., Gondivkar R., Gadbail A. et al. (2013) Chronic periodontitis and the risk of head and neck squamous cell carcinoma: facts and figures. *Experimental Oncology,* 35:163-167. PMID: 24084452

47. Han Y., Houcken W., Loos B. et al. (2014) Periodontal disease, atherosclerosis, adverse pregnancy outcomes, and head-and-neck cancer. *Advances in Dental Research,* 26:47-55. PMID: 24736704

48. Sato Y., Motoyama S., Takano H. et al. (2016) Esophageal cancer patients have a high incidence of severe periodontitis and preoperative dental care reduces the likelihood of severe pneumonia after esophagectomy. *Digestive Surgery,* 33:495-502. PMID: 27287475

49. Zeng X., Xia L., Zhang Y. et al. (2016) Periodontal disease and incident lung cancer risk: a meta-analysis of cohort studies. *Journal of Periodontology,* Jun 13:1-13 [Epub ahead of print]. PMID: 27294431

50. Harris S., Harris E. (2015) Herpes simplex virus type 1 and other pathogens are key causative factors in sporadic Alzheimer's disease. *Journal of Alzheimer's Disease,* 48:319-353. PMID: 26401998

51. Singhrao S., Harding A., Poole S. et al. (2015) *Porphyromonas gingivalis* periodontal infection and its putative links with Alzheimer's disease. *Mediators of Inflammation,* 2015:137357. PMID: 26063967

52. Olsen I., Singhrao S. (2015) Can oral infection be a risk factor for Alzheimer's disease? *Journal of Oral Microbiology,* 7:29143. PMID: 26385886

53. Ide M., Harris M., Stevens A. et al. (2016) Periodontitis and cognitive decline in Alzheimer's disease. *PLoS One,* 11:e0151081. PMID: 26963387

54. Miklossy J., McGeer P. (2016) Common mechanisms involved in Alzheimer's disease and type 2 diabetes: a key role of chronic bacterial infection and inflammation. *Aging*, 8:575-588. PMID: 26961231

55. Sparks Stein P., Steffen M., Smith C. et al. (2012) Serum antibodies to periodontal pathogens are a risk factor for Alzheimer's disease. *Alzheimer's & Dementia*, 8:196-203. PMID: 22546352

56. Noble J., Scarmeas N., Celenti R. et al. (2014) Serum IgG antibody levels to periodontal microbiota are associated with incident Alzheimer disease. *PLoS One*, 9:e114959. PMID: 25522313

57. Zenthofer A., Baumgart D., Cabrera T. et al. (2016) Poor dental hygiene and periodontal health in nursing home residents with dementia: an observational study. *Odontology*, May 9 [Epub ahead of print]. PMID: 27160268

58. Tang W., Sun F., Ungvari G., O'Donnell D. (2004) Oral health of psychiatric in-patients in Hong Kong. *The International Journal of Social Psychiatry*, 50:186-191. PMID: 15293435

59. Gopalakrishnapillai A., Iyer R., Kalantharakath T. (2012) Prevalence of periodontal disease among inpatients in a psychiatric hospital in India. *Special Care in Dentistry*, 32:196-204. PMID: 22943772

60. Kisely S. (2016) No mental health without oral health. *Canadian Journal of Psychiatry*, 61:277-282. PMID: 27254802

61. Yu Y., Kuo H. (2008) Association between cognitive function and periodontal disease in older adults. *Journal of the American Geriatrics Society*, 56:1693-1697. PMID: 18691281

62. Einarsdottir E., Gunnsteinsdottir H., Hallsdottir M. et al. (2016) Dental health of patients with Parkinson's disease in Iceland. *Special Care in Dentistry*, 29:123-127. PMID: 19938251

63. Muller T., Palluch R., Jackowski J. (2011) Caries and periodontal disease in patients with Parkinson's disease. *Special Care in Dentistry*, 31:178-181. PMID: 21950532

64. Kaur T., Uppoor A., Naik D. (2015) Parkinson's disease and periodontitis—the missing link? A review. *Gerodontology*, Feb 9 [Epub ahead of print]. PMID: 25664991

65. Kamer A., Fortea J., Videla S. et al. (2016) Periodontal disease's contribution to Alzheimer's disease progression in Down syndrome. *Alzheimer's & Dementia*, 2:49-57. PMID: 27239536

66. Bu X., Wang X., Xiang Y. et al. (2015) The association between infectious burden and Parkinson's disease: a case-control study. *Parkinsonism & Related Disorders*, 21:877-881. PMID: 26037459

67. Costa A., Yasuda C., Shibasaki W. et al. (2014) The association between periodontal disease and seizure severity in refractory epilepsy patients. *Seizure*, 23:227-230. PMID: 24456623

68. Hsu C., Hsu Y., Chen H. et al. (2015) Association of periodontitis and subsequent depression: a nationwide population-based study. *Medicine*, 94:e2347. PMID: 26705230

69. Dumitrescu A. (2016) Depression and inflammatory periodontal disease considerations—an interdisciplinary approach. *Frontiers in Psychology*, 7:347. PMID: 27047405

70. Sheu J., Lin H. (2013) Association between multiple sclerosis and chronic periodontitis: a population-based pilot study. *European Journal of Neurology*, 20:1053-1059. PMID: 23398363

71. Rodriguez Coyado M., Sanchez Temino V. (2015) [Periodontitis determining the onset and progression of Huntington's disease: review of the literature]. Article in Spanish. *Medwave*, 15:e6293. PMID: 26569646

72. de Souza C., Braosi A., Luczyszyn S. et al. (2014) Association among oral health parameters, periodontitis, and its treatment and mortality in patients undergoing hemodialysis. *Journal of Periodontology*, 85:e169-e178. PMID: 24224959

73. Chen Y., Shih C., Ou S. et al. (2015) Periodontal disease and risks of kidney function decline and mortality in older people: a community-based cohort study. *American Journal of Kidney Diseases*, 66:223-230. PMID: 25747403

74. Ricardo A., Athavale A., Chen J. et al. (2015) Periodontal disease, chronic kidney disease and mortality: results from the third National Health and Nutrition Examination Study. *BMC Nephrology*, 16:97. PMID: 26149680

75. Hansen G., Egeberg A., Holmstrup P., Hansen P. (2016) Relation of periodontitis to risk of cardiovascular and all-cause mortality (from a Danish Nationwide Cohort Study). *The American Journal of Cardiology*, 118:489-493. PMID: 27372888

76. Sharma P., Dietrich T., Ferro C. et al. (2016) Association between periodontitis and mortality in stages 3-5 chronic kidney disease: NHANES III and linked mortality study. *Journal of Clinical Periodontology*, 43:104-113. PMID: 26717883

77. Chrysanthakopoulos N., Chrysanthakopoulos P. (2016) Association between indices of clinically-defined periodontitis and self-reported history of systemic medical conditions. *Journal of Investigative and Clinical Dentistry*, 7:27-36. PMID: 25048420

78. Borgnakke W. (2015) Does treatment of periodontal disease influence systemic disease? *Dental Clinics of North America*, 59:885-917. PMID: 26427573

79. Renvert S., Pettersson T., Ohlsson O., Persson G. (2015) Bacterial profile and burden of periodontal infection in subjects with a diagnosis of acute coronary syndrome. *Journal of Periodontology*, 77:1110-1119. PMID: 16805672

80. Ruiz-Canela M., Bes-Rastrollo M., Martinez-Gonzalez M. (2016) The role of dietary inflammatory index in cardiovascular disease, metabolic syndrome and mortality. *International Journal of Molecular Sciences*, 17. PMID: 27527152

81. Khaw K., Bingham S., Welch A. et al. (2001) Relation between plasma ascorbic acid and mortality in men and women in EPIC-Norfolk prospective study: a prospective population study. European Prospective Investigation into Cancer and Nutrition. *Lancet*, 357:657-663. PMID: 11247548

82. Simon J., Hudes E., Tice J. (2001) Relation of serum ascorbic acid to mortality among US adults. *Journal of the American College of Nutrition*, 20:255-263. PMID: 11444422

83. Dashti-Khavidaki S., Talasaz A., Tabeefar H. et al. (2011) Plasma vitamin C concentrations in patients on routine hemodialysis and its relationship to patients' morbidity and mortality. *International Journal for Vitamin and Nutrition Research*, 81:197-203. PMID: 22237767

84. Goyal A., Terry M., Siegel A. (2013) Serum antioxidant nutrients, vitamin A, and mortality in U.S. adults. *Cancer Epidemiology, Biomarkers & Prevention*, 22:2202-2211. PMID: 23897583

85. Levy T. (2013) *Death by Calcium: Proof of the toxic effects of dairy and calcium supplements.* Henderson, NV: MedFox Publishing

86. D'Aiuto F., Sabbah W., Netuveli G. et al. (2008) Association of the metabolic syndrome with severe periodontitis in a large U. S. population-based survery. *The Journal of Clinical Endocrinology and Metabolism*, 93:3989-3994. PMID: 18682518

87. Furuta M., Shimazaki Y., Takeshita T. et al. (2013) Gender differences in the association between metabolic syndrome and periodontal disease: the Hisayama Study. *Journal of Clinical Peridontology*, 40:743-752. PMID: 23829196

88. Kaye E., Chen N., Cabral H. et al. (2016) Metabolic syndrome and periodontal disease progression in men. *Journal of Dental Research*, 95:822-828. PMID: 27025874

89. Levine R. (2013) Obesity, diabetes and periodontitis—a triangular relationship? *British Dental Journal*, 215:35-39. PMID: 23846063

90. El-Shinnawi U, Soory M. (2015) Actions of adjunctive nutritional antioxidants in periodontitis and prevalent systemic inflammatory diseases. Endocrine, *Metabolic & Immune Disorders Drug Targets*, 15:261-276. PMID: 25922082

91. Teshome A., Yitayeh A. (2016) The effect of periodontal therapy on glycemic control and fasting plasma glucose level in type 2 diabetic patients: systemic review and meta-analysis. *BMC Oral Health*, 17:31. PMID: 27473177

92. Khader Y., Khassawneh B., Obeidat B. et al. (2008) Periodontal status of patients with metabolic syndrome compared to those without metabolic syndrome. *Journal of Periodontology*, 79:2048-2053. PMID: 18980512

93. Fentoglu O., Sozen T., Oz S. et al. (2010) Short-term effects of periodontal therapy as an adjunct to anti-lipemic treatment. *Oral Diseases*, 16:648-654. PMID: 20412449

94. Sandi R., Pol K., Basavaraj P. et al. (2014) Association of serum cholesterol, trighyceride, high and low density lipoprotein (HDL and LDL) levels in chronic periodontitis subjects with risk for cardiovascular disease (CVD): a cross sectional study. *Journal of Clinical and Diagnostic Research*, 8:214-216. PMID: 24596778

95. Nicolosi L., Lewin P., Rudzinski J. et al. (2016) Relation between periodontal disease and arterial stiffness. *Journal of Periodontal Research*, Mar 28 [Epub ahead of print]. PMID: 27018040

96. Franek E., Napora M., Blach A. et al. (2010) Blood pressure and left ventricular mass in subjects with type 2 diabetes and gingivitis or chronic periodontitis. *Journal of Clinical Periodontology*, 37:875-880. PMID: 20796107

97. Umeizudike K., Ayanbadejo P., Onajole A. et al. (2016) Periodontal status and its association with self-reported hypertension in non-medical staff in a university teaching hospital in Nigeria. *Odonto-Stomatologie Tropicale*, 39:47-55. PMID:27434919

98. Ribeiro L., Santos J., Vieira C. et al. (2016) Association of dental infections with systemic diseases in Brazilian Native Indigenous: a cross-sectional study. *Journal of the American Society of Hypertension*, 10:413-419. PMID: 27039160

99. Leong X., Ng C., Badiah B., Das S. (2014) Association between hypertension and periodontitis: possible mechanisms. *TheScientificWorldJournal*, 2014:768237. PMID: 24526921

100. Soder P., Soder B., Nowak J., Jogestrand T. (2005) Early carotid atherosclerosis in subjects with periodontal disease. *Stroke*, 36:1195-1200. PMID: 15879347

101. Brun A., Range H., Prouvost B. et al. (2016) Intraplaque hemorrhage, a potential consequence of periodontal bacteria gathering in human carotid atherothrombosis. *Bulletin du Groupement International Pour la Recherche Scientifique en Stomatologie & Odontologie*, 53:e11. PMID: 27352423

102. Palm F., Lahdentausta L., Sorsa T. et al. (2014) Biomarkers of periodontitis and inflammation in ischemic stroke: a case-control study. *Innate Immunity*, 20:511-518. PMID: 24045341

103. Leira Y., Seoane J., Blanco M. et al. (2016) Association between periodontitis and ischemic stroke: a systemic review and meta-analysis. *European Journal of Epidemiology*, Jun 14 [Epub ahead of print]. PMID: 27300352

104. Leira Y., Lopez-Dequidt I., Arias S. et al. (2016) Chronic periodontitis is associated with lacunar infarct: a case-controlled study. *European Journal of Neurology*, Jul 15 [Epub ahead of print]. PMID: 27418418

105. Jimenez M., Krall E., Garcia R. et al. (2009) Periodontitis and incidence of cerebrovascular disease in men. *Annals of Neurology*, 66:505-512. PMID: 19847898

106. Slowik J., Wnuk M., Grzech K. et al. (2010) Periodontitis affects neurological deficit in acute stroke. *Journal of the Neurological Sciences*, 297:82-84. PMID: 20723913

107. Marques da Silva R., Caugant D., Eribe E. et al. (2006) Bacterial diversity in aortic aneurysms determined by 16S ribosomal RNA gene analysis. *Journal of Vascular Surgery*, 44:1055-1060. PMID: 17098542

108. Iwai T. (2009) Periodontal bacteremia and various vascular diseases. *Journal of Periodontal Research*, 44:689-694. PMID: 19874452

109. Ahn Y., Shin M., Han D. et al. (2016) Periodontitis is associated with the risk of subclinical atherosclerosis and peripheral arterial disease in Korean adults. *Atherosclerosis*, 251:311-318. PMID: 27450785

110. Igari K., Inoue Y., Iwai T. (2016) The epidemiologic and clinical findings of patients with Buerger disease. *Annals of Vascular Surgery*, 30:263-269. PMID: 26370744

111. Endo S., Mishima E., Takeuchi Y. et al. (2015) Periodontitis-associated septic pulmonary embolism caused by *Actinomyces* species identified by anaerobic culture of bronchoalveolar lavage fluid: a case report. *BMC Infectious Diseases*, 15:552. PMID: 26626753

112. Gomes-Filho I., de Oliveira T., da Cruz S. et al. (2014) Influence of periodontitis in the development of nosocomial pneumonia: a case control study. *Journal of Periodontology*, 85:e82-e90. PMID: 24171504

113. Dev Y., Goyal O. (2013) Recurrent lung infection due to chronic peri-odontitis. *Journal of the Indian Medical Association*, 111:127, 129. PMID: 24003573

114. Bansal M., Khatri M., Taneja V. (2013) Potential role of periodontal infection in respiratory diseases—a review. *Journal of Medicine and Life*, 6:244-248. PMID: 24155782

115. Usher A., Stockley R. (2013) The link between chronic periodontitis and COPD: a common role for the neutrophil? *BMC Medicine*, 11:241. PMID: 24229090

116. Si Y., Fan H., Song Y. et al. (2012) Association between periodontitis and chronic obstructive pulmonary disease in a Chinese population. *Journal of Periodontology*, 83:1288-1296. PMID: 22248220

117. Peter K., Mute B., Doiphode S. et al. (2013) Association between periodontal disease and chronic obstructive pulmonary disease: a reality or just a dogma? *Journal of Periodontology*, 84:1717-1723. PMID: 23339345

118. Chung J., Hwang H., Kim S., Kim T. (2016) Associations between periodontitis and chronic obstructive pulmonary disease: the 2010 to 2012 Korean National Health and Nutrition Examination Survey. *Journal of Periodontology*, 87:864-871. PMID: 26912338

119. Kucukcoskun M., Baser U., Oztekin G. et al. (2013) Initial periodontal treatment for prevention of chronic obstructive pulmonary disease exacerbations. *Journal of Periodontology*, 84:863-870. PMID: 23003917

120. Zhou X., Han J., Liu Z. et al. (2014) Effects of periodontal treatment on lung function and exacerbation frequency in patients with chronic obstructive pulmonary disease and chronic periodontitis: a 2-year pilot randomized controlled trial. *Journal of Clinical Periodontology*, 41:564-572. PMID: 24593836

121. Terashima T., Chubachi S., Matsuzake T. et al. (2016) The association between dental health and nutritional status in chronic obstructive pulmonary disease. *Chronic Respiratory Disease*, Apr 6 [Epub ahead of print]. PMID: 27056058

122. Gomes-Filho I., Soledade-Marques K., Seixas da Cruz S. et al. (2014) Does periodontal infection have an effect on severe asthma in adults? *Journal of Periodontology*, 85:e179-e187. PMID: 24224961

123. Chou Y., Lai K., Chen D. et al. (2015) Rheumatoid arthritis risk associated with periodontitis exposure: a nationwide, population-based cohort study. *PLoS One*, 10:e0139693. PMID: 26426533

124. Payne J., Golub L., Thiele G., Mikuls T. (2015) The link between periodontitis and rheumatoid arthritis: a periodontist's perspective. *Current Oral Health Reports*, 2:20-29. PMID: 25657894

125. Choi I., Kim J., Kim Y. et al. (2016) Periodontitis is associated with rheumatoid arthritis: a study with longstanding rheumatoid arthritis patients in Korea. *The Korean Journal of Internal Medicine*, Mar 25 [Epub ahead of print]. PMID: 27017391

126. Araujo V., Melo I., Lima V. (2015) Relationship between periodontitis and rheumatoid arthritis: review of the literature. *Mediators of Inflammation*, 2015:259074. PMID: 26347200

127. Venkataraman A., Almas K. (2015) Rheumatoid arthritis and periodontal disease. An update. *The New York State Dental Journal*, 81:30-36. PMID: 26521325

128. Correa J., Saraiva A., Queiroz-Junior C. et al. (2016) Arthritis-induced alveolar bone loss is associated with changes in the composition of oral microbiota. *Anaerobe*, 39:91-96. PMID: 26996070

129. Fuggle N., Smith T., Kaul A., Sofat N. (2016) Hand to mouth: a systematic review and meta-analysis of the association between rheumatoid arthritis and periodontitis. *Frontiers in Immunology*, 7:80. PMID: 26973655

130. Mikuls T., Thiele G., Deane K. et al. (2012) *Porphyromonas gingivalis* and disease-related autoantibodies in individuals at increased risk of rheumatoid arthritis. *Arthritis & Rheumatology*, 64:3522-3530. PMID: 22736291

131. Ogrendik M. (2013) Rheumatoid arthritis is an autoimmune disease caused by periodontal pathogens. *International Journal of General Medicine*, 6:383-386. PMID: 23737674

132. Mikuls T., Payne J., Yu F. et al. (2014) Periodontitis and *Porphyromonas gingivalis* in patients with rheumatoid arthritis. *Arthritis & Rheumatology*, 66:1090-1100. PMID: 24782175

133. Al-Katma M., Bissada N., Bordeaux J. et al. (2007) Control of periodontal infection reduces the severity of active rheumatoid arthritis. *Journal of Clinical Rheumatology*, 13:134-137. PMID: 17551378

134. Khare N., Vanza B., Sagar D. et al. (2016) Nonsurgical periodontal therapy decreases the severity of rheumatoid arthritis: a case-control study. *The Journal of Contemporary Dental Practice*, 17:484-488. PMID: 27484603

135. Silvestre F., Silvestre-Rangil J., Bagan L., Bagan J. (2016) Effect of nonsurgical periodontal treatment in patients with periodontitis and rheumatoid arthritis: a systemic review. *Medicina Oral, Patologia Oral y Cirugia Bucal*, 21:e349-e354. PMID: 26946202

136. Bello-Gualtero J., Lafaurie G., Hoyos L. et al. (2016) Periodontal disease in individuals with a genetic risk of developing arthritis and early rheumatoid arthritis: a cross-sectional study. *Journal of Periodontology*, 87:346-356. PMID: 26609697

137. Wendling D., Prati C. (2013) Spondyloarthritis and smoking: towards a new insight into the disease. *Expert Review of Clinical Immunology*, 9:511-516. PMID: 23730882

138. Coburn B., Sayles H., Payne J. et al. (2015) Performance of self-reported measures for periodontitis in rheumatoid arthritis and osteoarthritis. *Journal of Periodontology*, 86:16-26. PMID: 25269524

139. Egeberg A., Mallbris L., Gislason G. et al. (2016) Risk of periodontitis in patients with psoriasis and psoriatic arthritis. *Journal of the European Academy of Dermatology and Venereology*, Jul 21 [Epub ahead of print]. PMID: 27439545

140. Lange L., Thiele G., McCracken C. et al. (2016) Symptoms of periodontitis and antibody responses to *Porphyromonas gingivalis* in juvenile idiopathic arthritis. *Pediatric Rheumatology Online Journal*, 14:8. PMID: 26861944

141. Ehrlich G., Hu F., Sotereanos N. et al. (2014) What role do periodontal pathogens play in osteoarthritis and periprosthetic joint infections of the knee? *Journal of Applied Biomaterials & Functional Materials*, 12:13-20. PMID: 24921460

142. Zhang W., Swearingen E., Ju J. et al. (2010) *Porphyromonas gingivalis* invades osteoblasts and inhibits bone formation. *Microbes and Infection*, 12:838-845. PMID: 20538069

143. Herrera B., Bastos A., Coimbra L. et al. (2014) Peripheral blood mononuclear phagocytes from patients with chronic periodontitis are primed for osteoclast formation. *Journal of Periodontology*, 85:e72-e81. PMID: 24059638

144. Lopez-Lopez J., Castellanos-Cosano L., Estrugo-Devesa A. et al. (2015) Radiolucent periapical lesions and bone mineral density in post-menopausal women. *Gerodontology*, 32:195-201. PMID: 24164489

145. Straka M., Straka-Trapezanlidis M., Deglovic J., Varga I. (2015) Periodontitis and osteoporosis. *Neuro Endocrinology Letters*, 36:401-406. PMID: 26707036

146. Huang Y., Chang C., Liu S. et al (2016) The impact of oral hygiene maintenance on the association between periodontitis and osteoporosis: a nationwide population-based cross sectional study. *Medicine*, 95:e2348. PMID: 26871767

147. Penoni D., Leao A., Fernandes T., Torres S. (2016) Possible links between osteoporosis and periodontal disease. *Revista Brasileira de Reumatologia*, Feb 24 [Epub ahead of print]. PMID: 26973339

148. Richa R., Puranik M., Shrivastava A. (2016) Association between osteoporosis and periodontal disease among postmenopausal Indian women. *Journal of Investigative and Clinical Dentistry*, Jun 24 [Epub ahead of print]. PMID: 27339765

149. Segura-Egea J., Jimenez-Pinzon A., Rios-Santos J. et al. (2005) High prevalence of apical periodontitis amongst type 2 diabetic patients. *International Endodontic Journal*, 38:564-569. PMID: 16011776

150. Bullon P., Jaramillo R., Santos-Garcia R. et al. (2014) Relation of periodontitis and metabolic syndrome with gestational glucose metabolism disorder. *Journal of Periodontology*, 85:e1-e8. PMID: 23952077

151. Segura-Egea J., Martin-Gonzalez J., Cabanillas-Balsera D. et al. (2016) Association between diabetes and the prevalcnce of radiolucent periapical lesions in root-filled teeth: systematic review and meta-analysis. *Clinical Oral Investigations*, Apr 8 [Epub ahead of print]. PMID: 27055847

152. Tsao C., Darby I., Ebeling P. et al. (2013) Oral health risk factors for bisphosphonate-associated jaw osteonecrosis. *Journal of Oral and Maxillofacial Surgery*, 71:1360-1366. PMID: 23582590

153. Thumbigere-Math V., Michalowicz B., Hodges J. et al. (2014) Periodontal disease as a risk factor for bisphosphonate-related osteonecrosis of the jaw. *Journal of Periodontology*, 85:226-233. PMID: 23786404

154. Fernández Ayora A, et al, {2015) Dramatic osteonecrosis of the jaw associated with oral bisphosphonates, periodontitis, and dental implant removal. *J Clin Periodontol*. Feb;42(2):190-5. PMID: 25327450

155. Joshi N., Bissada N., Bodner D. et al. (2010) Association between periodontal disease and prostate-specific antigen levels in chronic prostatitis patients. *Journal of Periodontology*, 81:864-869. PMID: 20450358

156. Tenenbaum H., Mock D., Simor A. (1991) Periodontitis as an early presentation of HIV infection. *Canadian Medical Association Journal*, 144:1265-1269. PMID: 2025822

157. Moscicki A., Yao T., Ryder M. et al. (2016) The burden of oral disease among perinatally HIV-infected and HIV-exposed uninfected youth. *PLoS One*, 11:e0156459. PMID: 27299992

158. Valentine J., Saladyanant T., Ramsey K. et al. (2016) Impact of periodontal intervention on local inflammation, periodontitis, and HIV outcomes. *Oral Diseases*, Suppl 1:87-97. PMID: 27109277

159. Novo E., Garcia-MacGregor E., Viera N. et al. (1999) Periodontitis and anti-neutrophil cytoplasmic antibodies in systemic lupus erythematosus and rheumatoid arthritis: a comparative study. *Journal of Periodontology*, 70:185-188. PMID: 10102556

160. Schenkein H., Berry C., Burmeister J. et al. (2003) Anti-cardiolipin antibodies in sera from patients with periodontitis. *Journal of Dental Research*, 82:919-922. PMID: 14578506

161. Schenkein H., Best A., Brooks C. et al. (2007) Anti-cardiolipin and increased serum adhesion molecule levels in patients with aggressive periodontitis. *Journal of Periodontology*, 78:459-466. PMID: 17335369

162. Fabbri C., Fuller R., Bonfa E. et al. (2014) Periodontitis treatment improves systemic lupus erythematosus response to immunosuppressive therapy. *Clinical Rheumatology*, 33:505-509. PMID: 24415114

163. Marques C., Victor E., Franco M. et al. (2016) Salivary levels of inflammatory cytokines and their association to periodontal disease in systemic lupus erythematosus patients. A case-control study. *Cytokine*, 85:165-170. PMID: 27371775

164. Yadalam P., Rajapandian K., Ravishankar P. et al. (2016) Evaluation of anticardiolipin antibodies in tobacco users and non-tobacco users with severe chronic periodontal disease. *Journal of International Society of Preventive & Community Dentistry*, 6:256-260. PMID: 27382544

165. Pressman G., Qasim A., Verma N. et al. (2013) Periodontal disease is an independent predictor of intracardiac calcification. *BioMed Research International*, 2013:854340. PMID: 24106721

166. Bengtsson V., Persson G., Renvert S. (2014) Assessment of carotid calcifications on panoramic radiographs in relation to other used methods and relationship to periodontitis and stroke: a literature review. *Acta Odontologica Scandinavica*, 72:401-412. PMID: 24432815

167. Kamak G., Yildirim E., Rencber E. (2015) Evaluation of the relationship between periodontal risk and carotid artery calcifications on panoramic radiographs. *European Journal of Dentistry*, 9:483-489. PMID: 26929685

168. Bengtsson V., Persson G., Berglund J., Renvert S. (2016) A cross-sectional study of the associations between periodontitis and carotid arterial calcifications in an elderly population. *Acta Odontologica Scandinavica*, 74:115-120. PMID: 26066062

169. Liu Z., Liu Y., Song Y. et al. (2014) Systemic oxidative stress biomarkers in chronic periodontitis: a meta-analysis. *Disease Markers*, 2014:931083. PMID: 25477703

170. Brito F., de Barros F., Zaltman C. et al. (2008) Prevalence of periodontitis and DMFT index in patients with Crohn's disease and ulcerative colitis. *Journal of Clinical Periodontology*, 35:555-560. PMID: 18400026

171. Habashneh R., Khader Y., Alhumouz M. et al. (2012) The association between inflammatory bowel disease and periodontitis among Jordanians: a case-control study. *Journal of Periodontal Research*, 47:293-298. PMID: 22050539

172. Brito F., Zaltman C., Carvalho A. et al. (2013) Subgingival microflora in inflammatory bowel disease patients with untreated periodontitis. European *Journal of Gastroenterology & Hepatology*, 25:239-245. PMID: 23060013

173. Vavricka S., Manser C., Hediger S. et al. (2013) Periodontitis and gingivitis in inflammatory bowel disease: a case-control study. *Inflammatory Bowel Diseases*, 19:2768-2777. PMID: 24216685

174. Barak S., Oettinger-Barak O., Machtei E. et al. (2007) Evidence of peripathogenic microorganisms in placentas of women with preeclampsia. *Journal of Periodontology*, 78:670-676. PMID: 17397314

175. Alchalabi H., Al Habashneh R., Jabali O., Khader Y. (2013) Association between periodontal disease and adverse pregnancy outcomes in a cohort of pregnant women in Jordan. *Clinical and Experimental Obstetrics & Gynecology*, 40:399-402. PMID: 24283174

176. Chaparro A., Blanlot C., Ramirez V. et al. (2013) *Porphyromonas gingivalis, Treponema denticola* and toll-like receptor 2 are associated with hypertensive disorders in placental tissue: a case-control study. *Journal of Periodontal Research*, 48:802-809. PMID: 23711357

177. Jacob P., Nath S. (2014) Periodontitis among poor rural Indian mothers increases the risk of low birth weight babies: a hospital-based case control study. *Journal of Periodontal & Implant Science*, 44:85-93. PMID: 24778903

178. Kothiwale S., Desai B., Kothiwale V. et al. (2014) Periodontal disease as a potential risk factor for low birth weight and reduced maternal haemoglobin levels. *Oral Health & Preventive Dentistry*, 12:83-90. PMID: 24619787

179. Amarasekara R., Jayasekara R., Senanayake H., Dissanayake V. (2015) Microbiome of the placenta in pre-eclampsia supports the role of bacteria in the multifactorial cause of pre-eclampsia. *The Journal of Obstetrics and Gynaecology Research*, 41:662-669. PMID: 25492799

180. Lee H., Ha J., Bae K. (2016) Synergistic effect of maternal obesity and periodontitis on preterm birth in women with pre-eclampsia: a prospective study. *Journal of Clinical Periodontology*, 43:646-651. PMID: 27167920

181. Parihar A., Katoch V., Rajguru S. et al. (2016) Periodontal disease: a possible risk-factor for adverse pregnancy outcomes. *Journal of International Oral Health*, 7:137-142. PMID: 26229389

182. Anand P., Sagar D., Ashok S., Kamath K. (2014) Association of aggressive periodontitis with reduced erythrocyte counts and reduced hemoglobin levels. *Journal of Periodontal Research*, 49:719-728. PMID: 24329044

183. Kolte R., Kolte A., Desphande N. (2014) Assessment and comparison of anemia of chronic disease in healthy subjects and chronic periodontitis patients: a clinical and hematological study. *Journal of Indian Society of Periodontology*, 18:183-186. PMID: 24872626

184. Musalaiah S., Anupama M., Nagasree M. et al. (2014) Evaluation of nonsurgical periodontal therapy in chronic periodontitis patients with anemia by estimating hematological parameters and high-sensitivity C-reactive protein levels. *Journal of Pharmacy & Bioallied Sciences*, 6(Suppl 1):S64-S69. PMID: 25210388

185. Patel M., Shakir Q., Shetty A. (2014) Interrelationship between chronic periodontitis and anemia: a 6-month follow-up study. *Journal of Indian Society of Periodontology*, 18:19-25. PMID: 24744539

186. Khan N., Luke R., Soman R. et al. (2015) Qualitative assessment of red blood cell parameters for signs of anemia in patients with chronic periodontitis. *Journal of International Society of Preventive & Community Dentistry*, 5:476-481. PMID: 26759801

187. Salimi S., Ng N., Seliger S., Parsa A. (2014) Periodontal disease, renal dysfunction and heightened leukocytosis. *Nephron. Clinical Practice*. 128:107-114. PMID: 25402594

188. Ausavarungnirun R., Wisetsin S., Rongkiettechakorn N. et al. (2016) Association of dental and periodontal disease with chronic kidney disease in patients of a single, tertiary care centre in Thailand. *BMJ Open*, 6:e011836. PMID: 27466240

189. Wu C., Yang T., Lin H. et al. (2013) Sudden sensorineural hearing loss associated with chronic periodontitis: a population-based study. *Otology & Neurotology*, 34:1380-1384. PMID: 24026022

190. Sharma A., Pradeep A., Raju P. (2011) Association between chronic periodontitis and vasculogenic erectile dysfunction. *Journal of Periodontology*, 82:1665-1669. PMID: 21513476

191. Keller J., Chung S., Lin H. (2012) A nationwide population-based study on the association between chronic periodontitis and erectile dysfunction. *Journal of Clinical Periodontology*, 39:507-512. PMID: 22509774

192. Pussinen P., Tuomisto K., Jousilahti P. et al. (2007) Endotoxemia, immune response to periodontal pathogens, and systemic inflammation associate with incident cardiovascular disease events. *Arteriosclerosis, Thrombosis, and Vascular Biology*, 27:1433-1439. PMID: 17363692

193. Hayashi C., Gudino C., Gibson 3rd F., Genco C. (2010) Review: pathogen-induced inflammation at sites distant from oral infection: bacterial persistence and induction of cell-specific innate immune inflammatory pathways. *Molecular Oral Microbiology*, 25:305-316. PMID: 20883220

194. Gomes M., Blattner T., Sant'Ana Filho M. et al. (2013) Can apical periodontitis modify systemic levels of inflammatory levels? A systematic review and meta-analysis. *Journal of Endodontics*, 39:1205-1217. PMID: 24041380

195. Arregoces F., Uriza C., Porras J. et al. (2014) Relation between ultra-sensitive C-reactive protein, diabetes and periodontal disease in patients with and without myocardial infarction. *Arquivos Brasileiros de Endocrinologia e Metabologia*, 58:362-368. PMID: 24936730

196. Awang R., Lappin D., MacPherson A. et al. (2014) Clinical associations between IL-17 family cytokines and periodontitis and potential differential roles for IL-17A and IL-17E in periodontal immunity. *Inflammation Research*, 63:1001-1012. PMID: 25369802

197. Chakraborty S., Tewari S., Sharma R., Narula S. (2014) Effect of non-surgical periodontal therapy on serum ferritin levels: an interventional study. *Journal of Periodontology*, 85:688-696. PMID: 23826646

198. Liu Z., Liu Y., Song Y. et al. (2014) Systemic oxidative stress biomarkers in chronic periodontitis: a meta-analysis. *Disease Markers*, 2014:931083. PMID: 25477703

199. Sharma A., Astekar M., Metgud R. et al. (2014) A study of C-reactive protein, lipid metabolism and peripheral blood to identify a link between periodontitis and cardiovascular disease. *Biotechnic & Histochemistry*, 89:577-582. PMID: 24974939

200. El-Shinnawi U, Soory M. (2015) Actions of adjunctive nutritional antioxidants in periodontitis and prevalent systemic inflammatory diseases. *Endocrine, Metabolic & Immune Disorders Drug Targets*, 15:261-276. PMID: 25922082

Chapter 4

1. Kozlowski H., Kolkowska P., Watly J. et al. (2014) General aspects of metal toxicity. *Current Medicinal Chemistry*, 21:3721-3740. PMID: 25039781

2. Gozzelino R. (2016) The pathophysiology of heme in the brain. *Current Alzheimer Research*, 13:174-184. PMID: 26391040

3. Ikeda Y., Imao M., Satoh A. et al. (2016) Iron-induced skeletal muscle atrophy involves an Akt-forkhead box O3-E3 ubiquitin ligase-dependent pathway. *Journal of Trace Elements in Medicine and Biology*, 35:66-76. PMID: 27049128

4. Gutteridge J., Halliwell B. (1994) *Antioxidants in Nutrition, Health, and Disease.* New York, NY: Oxford University Press

5. Beckman K., Ames B. (1998) The free radical theory of aging matures. *Physiological Reviews,* 78:547-581. PMID: 9562038

6. Halliwell B. (2006) Reactive species and antioxidants. Redox biology is a fundamental theme of aerobic life. *Plant Physiology,* 141(2):312-322. PMID: 16760481

7. Stone I. (1972) *The Healing Factor. "Vitamin C" Against Disease.* New York, NY: Grosset & Dunlap

8. Levy T. (2002) *Curing the Incurable. Vitamin C, Infectious Diseases, and Toxins.* Henderson, NV: MedFox Publishing

9. Klenner F. (1954) Recent discoveries in the treatment of lockjaw with vitamin C and tolserol. *Tri-State Medical Journal,* July, pages 7-11.

10. Zickri M. (2014) Possible local stem cells activation by microcurrent application in experimentally injured soleus muscle. *International Journal of Stem Cells,* 7:79-86. PMID: 25473445

11. Fujiya H., Ogura Y., Ohno Y. et al. (2015) Microcurrent electrical neuromuscular stimulation facilitates regeneration of injured skeletal muscle in mice. *Journal of Sports Science & Medicine,* 14:297-303. PMID: 25983578

12. Brailoiu G., Brailoiu E. (2016) Modulation of calcium entry by the endo-lysosomal system. *Advances in Experimental Medicine and Biology,* 898:423-447. PMID: 27161239

13. Kim D., Nimigean C. (2016) Voltage-gated potassium channels: a structural examination of selectivity and gating. *Cold Spring Harbor Perspectives in Biology,* 8(5). PMID: 27141052

14. Sumikama T., (2016) Origin of the shape of current-voltage curve through nanopores: a molecular dynamics study. *Scientific Reports,* 6:25750. PMID: 27167118

15. Levy T. (2002) *Curing the Incurable. Vitamin C, Infectious Diseases, and Toxins.* Henderson, NV: MedFox Publishing

16. Meillier A., Heller C. (2015) Acute cyanide poisoning: hydroxocobalamin and sodium thiosulfate treatments with two outcomes following one exposure event. *Case Reports in Medicine,* 2015:217951. PMID: 26543483

17. Jia X., Cui J., Meng X. et al. (2016) Malignant transformation of human gastric epithelium cells via reactive oxygen species production and Wnt/β-catenin pathway activation following 40-week exposure to ochratoxin A. *Cancer Letters,* 372:36-47. PMID: 26721203

18. Santos C., Anilkumar N., Zhang M. et al. (2011) Redox signaling in cardiac myocytes. *Free Radical Biology & Medicine,* 50:777-793. PMID: 21236334

19. Abdul-Aziz A., MacEwan D., Bowles K., Rushworth S. (2015) Oxidative stress responses and NRF2 in human leukaemia. *Oxidative Medicine and Cellular Longevity,* 2015:454659. PMID: 25918581

20. Parri M., Chiarugi P. (2013) Redox molecular machines involved in tumor progression. *Antioxidants & Redox Signaling,* 19:1828-1845. PMID: 23146119

21. Zhou S., Liu R., Yuan K. et al. (2013) Proteomics analysis of tumor microenvironment: implications of metabolic and oxidative stresses in tumorigenesis. *Mass Spectrometry Reviews*, 32:267-311. PMID: 23165949

22. Kryston T., Georgiev A., Pissis P., Georgakilas A. (2011) Role of oxidative stress and DNA damage in human carcinogenesis. *Mutation Research*, 711(1-2):193-201. PMID: 21216256

23. Lin X., Zheng W., Liu J. et al. (2013) Oxidative stress in malignant melanoma enhances tumor necrosis factor-α secretion of tumor-associated macrophages that promote cancer cell invasion. *Antioxidants & Redox Signaling*, 19:1337-1355. PMID: 23373752

24. Sharma V., Joseph C., Ghosh S. et al. (2007) Kaempferol induces apoptosis in glioblastoma cells through oxidative stress. *Molecular Cancer Therapeutics*, 6:2544-2553. PMID: 17876051

25. Meshkini A., Yazdanparast R. (2012) Involvement of oxidative stress in taxol-induced apoptosis in chronic myelogenous leukemia K562 cells. *Experimental and Toxicologic Pathology*, 64:357-365. PMID: 21074392

Chapter 5

1. Terman A., Brunk U. (2006) Oxidative stress, accumulation of biological "garbage", and aging. *Antioxidants and Redox Signaling*, 8:197-204. PMID: 16487053

2. Gilca M., Stoian I., Atanasiu V., Virgolici B. (2007) The oxidative hypothesis of senescence. *Journal of Postgraduate Medicine*, 53:207-213. PMID: 17700000

3. Weber Jr F., Mitchell Jr G., Powell D. et al. (1982) Reversible hepatotoxicity associated with hepatic vitamin A accumulation in a protein-deficient patient. *Gastroenterology*, 82:118-123. PMID: 7198069

4. Snodgrass S. (1992) Vitamin neurotoxicity. *Molecular Neurobiology*, 6:41-73. PMID: 1463588

5. Sheth A., Khurana R., Krurana V. (2008) Potential liver damage associated with over-the-counter vitamin supplements. *Journal of the American Dietetic Association*, 108:1536-1537. PMID: 18755329

6. Allen S., Shah J. (1992) Calcinosis and metastatic calcification due to vitamin D intoxication. A case report and review. *Hormone Research*, 37(1-2):68-77. PMID: 1398478

7. Ginde A., Scragg R., Schwartz R., Camargo Jr C. (2009) Prospective study of serum 25-hydroxyvitamin D level, cardiovascular disease mortality, and all-cause mortality in older U.S. adults. *Journal of the American Geriatrics Society*, 57:1595-1603. PMID: 19549021

8. Semba R., Houston D., Bandinelli S. et al. (2010) Relationship of 25-hydroxyvitamin D with all-cause and cardiovascular mortality in older community-dwelling adults. *European Journal of Clinical Nutrition*, 64:203-209. PMID: 19953106

9. Bardosi A., Dickmann U. (1987) Necrotizing myopathy with paracrystalline inclusion bodies in hypervitaminosis E. *Acta Neuropathologica*, 75:166-172. PMID: 2829497

10. Sunder A., Halle I., Flachowsky G. (1999) Vitamin E hypervitaminosis in laying hens. *Archiv fur Tierernahrung*, 52:185-194. PMID: 10548970

11. Pucaj K., Rasmussen H., Moller M., Preston T. (2011) Safety and toxicological evaluation of a synthetic vitamin K2, menaquinone-7. *Toxicology Mechanisms and Methods*, 21:520-532. PMID: 21781006

12. McCarty M. (2000) Co-administration of equimolar doses of betaine may alleviate the hepatotoxic risk associated with niacin therapy. *Medical Hypotheses*, 55:189-194. PMID: 10985907

13. Tupe R., Tupe S., Agte V. (2011) Dietary nicotinic acid supplementation improves hepatic zinc uptake and offers hepatoprotection against oxidative damage. *The British Journal of Nutrition*, 105:1741-1749. PMID: 21262064

14. Ganji S., Kukes G., Lambrecht N. et al. (2014) Therapeutic role of niacin in the prevention and regression of hepatic steatosis in rat model of nonalcoholic fatty liver disease. *American Journal of Physiology. Gastrointestinal and Liver Physiology*, 306:G320-G327. PMID: 24356885

15. Rolfe H. (2014) A review of nicotinamide: treatment of skin diseases and potential side effects. *Journal of Cosmetic Dermatology*, 13:324-328. PMID: 25399625

16. Ghavanini A., Kimpinski K. (2014) Revisiting the evidence for neuropathy caused by pyridoxine deficiency and excess. *Journal of Clinical Neuromuscular Disease*, 16:25-31. PMID: 25137514

17. Kulkantrakorn K. (2014) Pyridoxine-induced sensory ataxic neuronopathy and neuropathy: revisited. *Neurological Sciences*, 35:1827-1830. PMID: 25056196

18. van der Watt J., Benatar M., Harrison T. et al. (2015) Isoniazid exposure and pyridoxine levels in human immunodeficiency virus associated distal sensory neuropathy. *The International Journal of Tuberculosis and Lung Disease*, 19:1312-1319. PMID: 26467583

19. Padayatty S., Sun A., Chen Q. et al. (2010) Vitamin C: intravenous use by complementary and alternative medicine practitioners and adverse effects. *PLoS One*, 5:e11414. PMID: 20628650

20. Kozler P., Pokorny J. (2014) CT density decrease in water intoxication rat model of brain oedema. *Neuro Endocrinology Letters*, 35:608-612. PMID: 25617884

21. Gill M., McCauley M. (2015) Psychogenic polydipsia: the result, or cause of, deteriorating psychotic symptoms? A case report of the consequences of water intoxication. *Case Reports in Psychiatry*, 2015:846459. PMID: 25688318

22. Lai J., Lu Q., Xu Y., Hu S. (2016) Severe water intoxication and secondary depressive syndrome in relation to delusional infestation. *Neuropsychiatric Disease and Treatment*, 12:517-521. PMID: 27013878

23. Losonczy L., Lovallo E., Schnorr C., Mantuani D. (2016) Drinking to near death—acute water intoxication leading to neurogenic stunned myocardium. *The American Journal of Emergency Medicine*, 34:119.e3-4. PMID: 26238098

24. Leone N., Courbon D., Ducimetiere P., Zureik M. (2006) Zinc, copper, and magnesium and risks for all-cause, cancer, and cardiovascular mortality. *Epidemiology*, 17:308-314. PMID: 16570028

25. Fardellone P., Cotte F., Roux C. et al. (2010) Calcium intake and the risk of osteoporosis and fractures in French women. *Joint, Bone, Spine* 77:154-158. PMID: 20185352

26. Sonneville K., Gordon C., Kocher M. et al. (2012) Vitamin D, calcium, and diary intakes and stress fractures among female adolescents. *Archives of Pediatrics & Adolescent Medicine*, 166:595-600. PMID: 22393172

27. Nasir K., Rubin J., Blaha M. et al. (2012) Interplay of coronary artery calcification and traditional risk factors for the prediction of all-cause mortality in asymptomatic individuals. Circulation. *Cardiovascular Imaging*, 5:467-473. PMID: 22718782

28. Michaelsson K., Melhus H., Warensjo Lemming E. et al. (2013) Long term calcium intake and rates of all cause and cardiovascular mortality: community based prospective longitudinal cohort study. BMJ, 346:f228. PMID: 23403980

29. Gillman M., Ross-Degnan D., McLaughlin T. et al. (1999) Effects of long-acting versus short-acting calcium channel blockers among older survivors of acute myocardial infarction. *Journal of the American Geriatrics Society*, 47:512-517. PMID: 10323641

30. Gibson R., Hansen J., Messerli F. et al. (2000) Long-term effects of diltiazem and verapamil on mortality and cardiac events in non-Q-wave acute myocardial infarction without pulmonary congestion: post hoc subset analysis of the multicenter diltiazem postinfarction trial and the second Danish verapamil infarction trial studies. *The American Journal of Cardiology*, 86:275-279. PMID: 10922432

31. Costanzo P., Perrone-Filardi P., Petretta M. et al. (2009) Calcium channel blockers and cardiovascular outcomes: a meta-analysis of 175,634 patients. *Journal of Hypertension*, 27:1135-1151. PMID: 19451836

32. Levy T. (2013) *Death by Calcium. Proof of the toxic effects of diary and calcium supplements.* Henderson, NV: MedFox Publishing

33. Gutteridge J., Halliwell B. (1994) *Antioxidants in Nutrition, Health, and Disease.* New York, NY: Oxford University Press

34. Kehrer J. (2000) The Haber-Weiss reaction and mechanisms of toxicity. *Toxicology*, 149:43-50. PMID: 10963860

35. Rivera-Mancia S., Perez-Neri I., Rios C. et al. (2010) The transition metals copper and iron in neurodegenerative diseases. *Chemico-Biological Interactions*, 186:184-199. PMID: 20399203

36. Kell D. (2010) Towards a unifying, systems biology understanding of large-scale cellular death and destruction caused by poorly liganded iron: Parkinson's, Huntington's, Alzheimer's, prions, bactericides, chemical toxicology and others as examples. *Archives of Toxicology*, 84:825-829. PMID: 20967426

37. Toyokuni S. (2016) The origin and future of oxidative stress pathology: from the recognition of carcinogenesis as an iron addiction with ferroptosis-resistance to nonthermal plasma therapy. *Pathology International*, 66:245-259. PMID: 26931176

38. Richardson D. (2002) Therapeutic potential of iron chelators in cancer therapy. *Advances in Experimental Medicine and Biology*, 509:231-249. PMID: 12572997

39. Salonen J., Nyyssonen K., Korpela H. et al. (1992) High stored iron levels are associated with excess risk of myocardial infarction in eastern Finnish men. *Circulation*, 86:803-811. PMID: 1516192
40. Rowland T., Black S., Kelleher J. (1987) Iron deficiency in adolescent endurance athletes. *Journal of Adolescent Health Care*, 8:322-326. PMID: 3610736
41. Zheng H., Cable R., Spencer C. et al. (2005) Iron stores and vascular function in voluntary blood donors. *Arteriosclerosis, Thrombosis, and Vascular Biology*, 25:1577-1583. PMID: 15961703
42. Fuchs A., Mariotto R., de Lustig E. (1986) Serum and tissue copper content in two mammary adenocarcinomas with different biological behaviour. *European Journal of Cancer & Clinical Oncology*, 22:1347-1352. PMID: 3830216
43. Fuchs A., de Lustig E. (1989) Localizations of tissue copper in mouse mammary tumors. *Oncology*, 46:183-187. PMID: 2470002
44. Liu X. (1991) [Serum and tissue copper, zinc and selenium levels in patients with gastric carcinoma]. Article in Chinese. *Zhonghua Zhong Liu Za Zhi (Chinese Journal of Oncology)*, 13:93-96. PMID: 1879301
45. Gupta S., Shukla V., Vaidya M. et al. (1993) Serum and tissue trace elements in colorectal cancer. *Journal of Surgical Oncology*, 52:172-175. PMID: 8441275
46. Yoshida D., Ikeda Y., Nakazawa S. (1993) Quantitative analysis of copper, zinc and copper/zinc ratio in selected human brain tumors. *Journal of Neuro-Oncology*, 16:109-115. PMID: 8289088
47. Gupta S., Singh S., Shukla V. (2005) Copper, zinc, and Cu/Zn ratio in carcinoma of the gallbladder. *Journal of Surgical Oncology*, 91:204-208. PMID: 16118778
48. Chen D., Dou Q. (2008) New uses for old copper-binding drugs: converting the pro-angiogenic copper to a specific cancer cell death inducer. *Expert Opinion on Therapeutics Targets*, 12:739-748. PMID: 18479220
49. Mizukami S., Ichimura R., Kemmochi S. et al. (2010) Tumor promotion by copper-overloading and its enhancement by excess iron accumulation involving oxidative stress responses in the early stage of a rat two-stage hepatocarcinogenesis model. *Chemico-Biological Interactions*, 185:189-201. PMID: 20302851
50. Rigiracciolo D., Scarpelli A., Lappano R. et al. (2015) Copper activates HIP-1α/GPER/VEGF signalling in cancer cells. *Oncotarget*, 6:34158-34177. PMID: 26415222
51. Salonen J., Salonen R., Korpela H. et al. (1991) Serum copper and the risk of acute myocardial infarction: a prospective population study in men in Eastern Finland. *American Journal of Epidemiology*, 134:268-276. PMID: 1877585
52. Stadler N., Lindner R., Davies M. (2004) Direct detection and quantification of transition metal ions in human atherosclerotic plaques: evidence for the presence of elevated levels of iron and copper. *Arteriosclerosis, Thrombosis, and Vascular Biology*, 24:949-954. PMID: 15001454

53. Ellervik C., Marott J., Tybjaerg-Hansen A. et al. (2014) Total and cause-specific mortality by moderately and markedly increased ferritin concentrations: general population study and metaanalysis. *Clinical Chemistry*, 60:1419-1428. PMID: 25156997

54. Malavolta M., Giacconi R., Piacenza F. et al. (2010) Plasma copper/zinc ratio: an inflammatory/nutritional biomarker as predictor of all-cause mortality in elderly population. *Biogerontology*, 11:309-319. PMID: 19821050

55. Wisner F. (1925) Focal infection, a medico-dental problem. *California and Western Medicine*, 23:977-980. PMID: 18739726

56. Kolmer J. (1950) Focal infection in the etiology of disease. *Journal of the National Medical Association*, 42:1-7. PMID: 15398955

57. Pentecost R. (1922) Focal infection in the tonsils of adults suffering from sub-acute and chronic systemic disease. Analysis of results of removal in a series of 800 cases. The *Canadian Medical Association Journal*, 12:886-891. PMID: 20314268

58. Leslie-Roberts H. (1922) Focal infection in relation to the etiology of skin diseases. *The British Medical Journal*, 1(3190):262-264. PMID: 20770602

59. Billings F. (1930) Focal infection as the cause of general disease. *Bulletin of the New York Academy of Medicine*, 12:759-773. PMID: 19311755

60. Auld J. (1927) Focal infection in relation to systemic disease. *The Canadian Medical Association Journal*, 17:294-297. PMID: 20316215

61. Nakamura T. (1929) A study on focal infection and elective localization in ulcer of the stomach and in arthritis. *Annals of Surgery*, 79:29-43. PMID: 17864965

62. Daland J. (1922) Diagnosis of focal infection. *Transactions of the American Climatological and Clinical Association*, 38:66-71. PMID: 21408811

63. Cecil R. (1934) Focal infection—some modern aspects. *California and Western Medicine*, 40:397-403. PMID: 18742882

64. Henry C. (1920) Focal infection. *The Canadian Medical Association Journal*, 10:593-604. PMID: 20312306

65. Wilkins T., Embry K., George R. (2013) Diagnosis and management of acute diverticulitis. *American Family Physician*, 87:612-620. PMID: 23668524

66. Pfutzer R., Kruis W. (2015) Management of diverticular disease. *Nature Reviews. Gastroenterology & Hepatology*, 12:629-638. PMID: 26170219

67. Lee Y., Erdogan A., Rao S. (2014) How to assess regional and whole gut transit time with wireless motility capsule. *Journal of Neurogastroenterology and Motility*, 20:265-270. PMID: 24840380

68. Roland B., Ciarleglio M., Clarke J. et al. (2015) Small intestinal transit time is delayed in small intestinal bacterial overgrowth. *Journal of Clinical Gastroenterology*, 49:571-576. PMID: 25319735

69. Lin J., Lin C., Yang C. et al. (2015) Increased risk of acute coronary syndrome in patients with diverticular disease: a nationwide population-based study. *Medicine*, 94:e2020. PMID: 26559302

70. Tian H., Ding C., Gong J. et al. (2016) Treatment of slow transit constipation with fecal microbiota transplantation: a pilot study. *Journal of Clinical Gastroenterology*, Jan 8. PMID: 26751143

71. Levy T. (2001) *Optimal Nutrition for Optimal Health*. New York, NY: Keats Publishing

72. Weinberg E. (2009) Iron availability and infection. *Biochimica et Biophysica Acta*, 1790:600-605. PMID: 18675317

73. Gordeuk V., Brittenham G., McLaren G., Spagnuolo P. (1986) Hyperferremia in immunosuppressed patients with acute nonlymphocytic leukemia and the risk of infection. *The Journal of Laboratory and Clinical Medicine*, 108:466-472. PMID: 3534124

74. Halliwell B., Aruoma O., Mufti G., Bomford A. (1988) Bleomycin-detectable iron in serum from leukaemic patients before and after chemotherapy. Therapeutic implications for treatment with oxidant-generating drugs. *FEBS Letters*, 241:202-204. PMID: 2461877

75. Harrison P., Marwah S., Hughes R., Bareford D. (1994) Non-transferrin bound iron and neutropenia after cytotoxic chemotherapy. *Journal of Clinical Pathology*, 47:350-352. PMID: 8027374

76. Drakesmith H., Prentice A. (2008) Viral infection and iron metabolism. *Nature Reviews. Microbiology*, 6:541-552. PMID: 18552864

77. Khaw K., Dowsett M., Folkerd E. et al. (2007) Endogenous testosterone and mortality due to all causes, cardiovascular disease, and cancer in men: European prospective investigation into cancer in Norfolk (EPIC-Norfolk) Prospective Population Study. *Circulation*, 116:2694-2701. PMID: 18040028

78. Laughlin G., Barrett-Connor E., Bergstrom J. (2008) Low serum testosterone and mortality in older men. *The Journal of Clinical Endocrinology and Metabolism*, 93:68-75. PMID: 17911176

79. Vikan T., Schirmer H. Njolstad I., Svartberg (2009) Endogenous sex hormones and the prospective association with cardiovascular disease and mortality in men: the Tromso Study. *European Journal of Endocrinology*, 161:435-442. PMID: 19542243

80. Fukai S., Akishita M., Yamada S. et al. (2011) Plasma sex hormone levels and mortality in disabled older men and women. *Geriatrics & Gerontology International*, 11:196-203. PMID: 21143567

81. de Padua Mansur A., Silva T., Takada J. et al. (2012) Long-term prospective study of the influence of estrone levels on events in postmenopausal women with or at high risk for coronary artery disease. *TheScientificWorldJournal*, 2012:363595. PMID: 22701354

82. Grossmann M., Hoermann R., Gani L. et al. (2012) Low testosterone levels as an independent predictor of mortality in men with chronic liver disease. *Clinical Endocrinology*, 77:323-328. PMID: 22280063

83. Pereg D., Tirosh A., Elis A. et al. (2012) Mortality and coronary heart disease in euthyroid patients. *The American Journal of Medicine*, 125:826.e7-12. PMID: 22608790

84. Yang J., Han S., Song S. et al. (2012) Serum T3 level can predict cardiovascular events and all-cause mortality rates in CKD patients with proteinuria. *Renal Failure*, 34:364-372. PMID: 22260378

85. Rhee C., Alexander E., Bhan I., Brunelli S. (2013) Hypothyroidism and mortality among dialysis patients. *Clinical Journal of the American Society of Nephrology*, 8:593-601. PMID: 23258793

86. Tivesten A., Vandenput L., Labrie F. et al. (2009) Low serum testosterone and estradiol predict mortality in elderly men. *The Journal of Clinical Endocrinology and Metabolism*, 94:2482-2488. PMID: 19401373

87. Tseng F., Lin W., Lin C. et al. (2012) Subclinical hypothyroidism is associated with increased risk for all-cause and cardiovascular mortality in adults. *Journal of the American College of Cardiology*, 60:730-737. PMID: 22726629

88. Ceresini G., Ceda G., Lauretani F. et al. (2013) Thyroid status and 6-year mortality in elderly people living in a mildly iodine-deficient area: the aging in the Chianti Area Study. *Journal of the American Geriatric Society*, 61:868-874. PMID: 23647402

89. Schairer C., Adami H., Hoover R., Persson I. (1997) Cause-specific mortality in women receiving hormone replacement therapy. *Epidemiology*, 8:59-65. PMID: 9116097

90. Alexandersen P., Tanko L., Bagger Y. et al. (2006) The long-term impact of 2-3 years of hormone replacement therapy on cardiovascular mortality and atherosclerosis in healthy women. *Climacteric*, 9:108-118. PMID: 16698657

91. Pessi T., Karhunen V, Karjalainen P. et al. (2013) Bacterial signatures in thrombus aspirates of patients with myocardial infarction. *Circulation*, 127:1219-1228. PMID: 23418311

92. Barnes B., Galton L. (1976) *Hypothyroidism: The Unsuspected Illness*. New York, NY: Harper & Row

93. Tevaarwerk G. (2014) Two patients with atypical low triiodothyronine syndrome: primary deiodinase abnormalities? *Endocrinology, Diabetes & Metabolism Case Reports*, 2014:130055. PMID: 24683478

94. Mancini A., Di Segni C., Raimondo S. et al. (2016) Thyroid hormones, oxidative stress, and inflammation. *Mediators of Inflammation*, 2016:6757154. PMID: 27051079

95. Maia A., Kim B., Huang S. et al. (2005) Type 2 iodothyronine deiodinase is the major source of plasma T3 in euthyroid humans. *The Journal of Clinical Investigation*, 115:2524-2533. PMID: 16127464

96. Chopra I. (1997) Clinical review 86: Euthyroid sick syndrome: is it a misnomer? *The Journal of Clinical Endocrinology and Metabolism*, 82:329-334. PMID: 9024211

Chapter 6

1. Kulacz R., Levy T. (2014) *The Toxic Tooth: How a root canal could be making you sick*. Henderson, NV: MedFox Publishing

2. Siqueira Jr. J., Rocas I. (2009) Diversity of endodontic microbiota revisited. *Journal of Dental Research*, 88:969-981. PMID: 19828883

3. Nobrega L., Delboni M., Martinho F. et al. (2013) *Treponema* diversity in root canals with endodontic failure. *European Journal of Dentistry*, 7:61-68. PMID: 23408792

4. Antunes H., Rocas I., Alves F., Siqueira Jr. J. (2015) Total and specific bacterial levels in the apical root canal system of teeth with post-treatment apical periodontitis. *Journal of Endodontics*, 41:1037-1042. PMID: 25892512

5. Vidana R., Sullivan A., Billstrom H. et al. (2011) *Enterococcus faecalis* infection in root canals—host-derived or exogenous source? *Letters in Applied Microbiology*, 52:109-115. PMID: 21155997

6. Martinho F., Chiesa W., Zaia A. et al. (2011) Comparison of endotoxin levels in previous studies on primary endodontic infections. *Journal of Endodontics*, 37:163-167. PMID: 21238796

7. Gomes B., Endo M., Martinho F. (2012) Comparison of endotoxin levels found in primary and secondary endodontic infections. *Journal of Endodontics*, 38:1082-1086. PMID: 22794210

8. Waltimo T., Sen B., Meurman J. et al. (2003) Yeasts in apical periodontitis. *Critical Reviews in Oral Biology and Medicine*, 14:128-137. PMID: 12764075

9. Nair P., Pajarola G., Schroeder H. (1996) Types and incidence of human periapical lesions obtained with extracted teeth. *Oral Surgery, Oral Medicine, Oral Pathology, Oral Radiiology, and Endodontics*, 81:93-102. PMID: 8850492

10. Siqueira Jr. J., Rocas I. (2007) Bacterial pathogenesis and mediators in apical periodontitis. *Brazilian Dental Journal*, 18:267-280. PMID: 18278296

11. Siqueira Jr. J., Rocas I. (2013) Microbiology and treatment of acute apical abscesses. *Clinical Microbiology Reviews*, 26:255-273. PMID: 23554416

12. Jakovljevic A., Andric M., Knezevic A. et al. (2015) Human cytomegalovirus and Epstein-Barr virus genotypes in apical periodontitis lesions. *Journal of Endodontics*, 41:1847-1851. PMID: 26435468

13. Hernandez Vigueras S., Donoso Zuniga M., Jane-Salas E. et al. (2016) Viruses in pulp and periapical inflammation: a review. *Odontology*, 104:184-191. PMID: 25796386

14. Hommez G., De Meerleer G., De Neve W., De Moor R. (2012) Effect of radiation dose on the prevalence of apical periodontitis—a dosimetric analysis. *Clinical Oral Investigations*, 16:1543-1547. PMID: 22219024

15. Nair P. (2004) Pathogenesis of apical periodontitis and the causes of endodontic failures. *Critical Reviews in Oral Biology and Medicine*, 15:348-381. PMID: 15574679

16. Garcia C., Sempere F., Diago M., Bowen E. (2007) The post-endodontic periapical lesion: histologic and etiopathogenic aspects. *Medicina Oral, Patologia Oral Y Cirugia Bucal*, 12:E585-E590. PMID: 18059244

17. Siqueira Jr. J., Rocas I. (2007) Bacterial pathogenesis and mediators in apical periodontitis. *Brazilian Dental Journal*, 18:267-280. PMID: 18278296

18. Muliyar S., Shameem K., Thankachan R. et al. (2014) Microleakage in endodontics. *Journal of International Oral Health*, 6:99-104. PMID: 25628496

19. Petersen J., Glasl E., Nasseri P. et al. (2014) The association of chronic apical periodontitis and endodontic therapy with atherosclerosis. *Clinical Oral Investigations*, 18:1813-1823. PMID: 24338091

20. Gomes M., Hugo F., Hilgert J. et al. (2016) Apical periodontitis and incident cardiovascular events in the Baltimore Longitudinal Study of Ageing. *International Endodontic Journal*, 49:334-342. PMID: 26011008

21. Liljestrand J., Mantyla P., Paju S. et al. (2016) Association of endodontic lesions with coronary artery disease. *Journal of Dental Research*, Jul 27 [Epub ahead of print]. PMID: 27466397

22. Cardoso F., Ferreira N., Martinho F. et al. (2015) Correlation between volume of apical periodontitis determined by cone-beam computed tomography analysis and endotoxin levels found in primary root canal infection. *Journal of Endodontics*, 41:1015-1019. PMID: 25935504

23. Costa A., Yasuda C., Shibasaki W. et al. (2014) The association between periodontal disease and seizure severity in refractory epilepsy patients. *Seizure*, 23:227-230. PMID: 24456623

24. An G., Morse D., Kunin M. et al. (2016) Association of radiographically diagnosed apical periodontitis and cardiovascular disease: a hospital records-based study. *Journal of Endodontics*, 42:916-920. PMID: 27091354

25. Pessi T., Karhunen V, Karjalainen P. et al. (2013) Bacterial signatures in thrombus aspirates of patients with myocardial infarction. *Circulation*, 127:1219-1228. PMID: 23418311

26. Caplan D. (2014) Chronic apical periodontitis is more common in subjects with coronary artery disease. *The Journal of Evidence-Based Dental Practice*, 14:149-150. PMID: 25234220

27. Shaw L., Harjunmaa U., Doyle R. et al. (2016) Distinguishing the signals of gingivitis and periodontitis in supragingival plaque: a cross-sectional cohort study in Malawi. *Applied and Environmental Microbiology*, Aug 12 [Epub ahead of print]. PMID: 27520811

28. Segura-Egea J., Castellanos-Cosano L., Machuca G. et al. (2012) Diabetes mellitus, periapical inflammation and endodontic treatment outcome. *Medicina Oral, Patologia Oral y Cirugia Bucal*, 17:e356-e361. PMID: 22143698

29. Razi T., Mohammadi A., Ghojazadeh M. (2012) Comparison of accuracy of conventional periapical radiography and direct digital subtraction radiography with or without image enhancement in the diagnosis of density changes. *Journal of Dental Research, Dental Clinics, Dental Prospects,* 6:54-58. PMID: 22991637

30. Kanagasingam S., Hussaini H., Soo I. et al. (2016) Accuracy of single and parallax film and digital periapical radiographs in diagnosing apical periodontitis—a cadaver study. *International Endodontic Journal,* Apr 11 [Epub ahead of print]. PMID: 27063356

31. Estrela C., Leles C., Hollanda A. et al. (2008) Prevalence and risk factors of apical periodontitis in endodontically treated teeth in a selected population of Brazilian adults. *Brazilian Dental Journal,* 19:34-39. PMID: 18438557

32. Lofthag-Hansen S., Huumonen S., Grondahl K., Grondahl H. (2007) Limited cone-beam CT and intraoral radiography for the diagnosis of periapical pathology. *Oral Surgery, Oral Medicine, Oral Pathology, Oral Radiology, and Endodontics,* 103:114-119. PMID: 17178504

33. Davies A., Mannocci F., Mitchell P. et al. (2015) The detection of periapical pathoses in root filled teeth using single and parallax periapical radiographs versus cone beam computed tomography—a clinical study. *International Endodontic Journal,* 48:582-592. PMID: 25074727

34. Leonardi Dutra K., Haas L., Porporatti A. et al. (2016) Diagnostic accuracy of cone-beam computed tomography and conventional radiography on apical periodontitis: a systemic review and meta-analysis. *Journal of Endodontics,* 42:356-364. PMID: 26902914

35. Saidi A., Naaman A., Zogheib C. (2015) Accuracy of cone-beam computed tomography and periapical radiography in endodontically treated teeth evaluation: a five-year retrospective study. *Journal of International Oral Health,* 7:15-19. PMID: 25878472

36. Estrela C., Bueno M., Azevedo B. et al. (2008a) A new periapical index based on cone beam computed tomography. *Journal of Endodontics,* 34:1325-1331. PMID: 18928840

37. Venskkutonis T., Daugela P., Strazdas M., Juodzbalys G. (2014) Accuracy of digital radiography and cone beam computed tomography on periapical radiolucency detection in endodontically treated teeth. *Journal of Oral & Maxillofacial Research,* 5:e1. PMID: 25089173

38. von Arx T., Janner S., Hanni S., Bornstein M. (2015) Agreement between 2D and 3D radiographic outcome assessment one year after periapical surgery. *International Endodontic Journal,* Sep 9 [Epub ahead of print]. PMID: 26356580

39. Davies A., Patel S., Foschi F. et al. (2016) The detection of periapical pathoses using digital periapical radiography and cone beam computed tomography in endodontically retreated teeth—part 2: a 1 year post-treatment follow-up. *International Endodontic Journal,* 49:623-635. PMID: 26174351

40. de Paula-Silva F., Wu M., Leonardo M. et al. (2009) Accuracy of periapical radiography and cone-beam computed tomography scans in diagnosing apical periodontitis using histopathological findings as a gold standard. *Journal of Endodontics*, 35:1009-1012. PMID: 19567324

41. Gumru B., Tarcin B., Iriboz E. et al. (2015) Assessment of the periapical health of abutment teeth: a retrospective radiological study. *Nigerian Journal of Clinical Practice*, 18:472-476. PMID: 25966717

42. Haheim L., Olsen I., Ronningen K. (2011) Association between tooth extraction due to infection and myocardial infarction. *Community Dentistry and Oral Epidemiology*, 39:393-397. PMID: 21557755

43. Spivakovsky S. (2012) Myocardial infarction and tooth extraction associated. *Evidence-Based Dentistry*, 13:110. PMID: 23258177

44. Brasil S., Santos R., Fernandes A. et al. (2016) Influence of estrogen deficiency on the development of apical periodontitis. *International Endodontic Journal*, Jan 28 [Epub ahead of print]. PMID: 26821330

45. Garrido M., Dezerega A., Bordagaray M. et al. (2015) C-reactive protein expression is up-regulated in apical lesions of endodontic origin in association with interleukin-6. *Journal of Endodontics*, 41:464-469. PMID: 25748492

46. Vidal F., Fontes T., Marques T., Goncalves L. (2015) Association between apical periodontitis lesions and plasmatic levels of C-reactive protein, interleukin 6 and fibrinogen in hypertensive patients. *International Endodontic Journal*, Oct 24 [Epub ahead of print]. PMID: 26499471

47. Zhang J., Huang X., Lu B. et al. (2015) Can apical periodontitis affect serum levels of CRP, IL-2, and IL-6 as well as induce pathological changes in remote organs? *Clinical Oral Investigations*, Nov 10 [Epub ahead of print]. PMID: 26556576

48. Cintra L., Samuel R., Azuma M. et al. (2016) Multiple apical periodontitis influences serum levels of cytokines and nitric oxide. *Journal of Endodontics*, 42:747-751. PMID: 27059651

49. Ma N., Qu L., Xu L. et al. (2016) [Expression of IL-34 in chronic periapical lesions and its clinical significance]. Article in Chinese. *Shanghai Kou Qiang Yi Xue*, 25:53-57. PMID: 27063309

50. Kakehashi S., Stanley H., Fitzgerald R. (1965) The effects of surgical exposures of dental pulps in germ-free and conventional laboratory rats. *Oral Surgery, Oral Medicine, and Oral Pathology*, 20:340-349. PMID: 14342926

51. Siqueira Jr. J. (2002) Endodontic infections: concepts, paradigms, and perspectives. *Oral Surgery, Oral Medicine, Oral Pathology, Oral Radiology, and Endodontics*, 94:281-293. PMID: 12324780

52. Fabricius L., Dahlen G., Holm S., Moller A. (1982) Influence of combinations of oral bacteria on periapical tissues of monkeys. *Scandinavian Journal of Dental Research*, 90:200-206. PMID: 7051261

53. Moller A., Fabricius L., Dahlen G. et al. (2004) Apical periodontitis development and bacterial response to endodontic treatment. Experimental root canal infections in monkeys with selected bacterial strains. *European Journal of Oral Sciences*, 112:207-215. PMID: 15154917

54. Nair P., Pajarola G., Schroeder H. (1996) Types and incidence of human periapical lesions obtained with extracted teeth. *Oral Surgery, Oral Medicine, Oral Pathology, Oral Radiiology, and Endodontics*, 81:93-102. PMID: 8850492

Chapter 7

1. Scadding G. (1990) Immunology of the tonsil: a review. *Journal of the Royal Society of Medicine*, 83:104-107. PMID: 2181132

2. Issels J. (1999) *Cancer, A Second Opinion*, Garden City Park, NY: Avery Publishing Group

3. Nair P. (2004) Pathogenesis of apical periodontitis and the causes of endodontic failures. *Critical Reviews in Oral Biology and Medicine*, 15:348-381. PMID: 15574679

4. Hoddeson E., Gourin C. (2009) Adult tonsillectomy: current indications and outcomes. *Otolaryngology—Head and Neck Surgery*, 140:19-22. PMID: 19130955

Chapter 8

1. Murray C., Thomson W., Leichter J. (2016) Dental implant use in New Zealand: a 10-year update. *The New Zealand Dental Journal*, 112:49-54. PMID: 27506001

2. Adell R., Lekholm U., Rockler B., Branemark P. (1981) A 15-year study of osseointegrated implants in the treatment of the edentulous jaw. *International Journal of Oral Surgery*, 10:387-416. PMID: 6809663

3. Bosshardt D., Chappuis V., Buser D. (2017) Osseointegration of titanium, titanium alloy and zirconia dental implants: current knowledge and open questions. *Periodontology 2000*, 73:22-40. PMID: 28000277

4. Valente N., Andreana S. (2016) Peri-implant disease: what we know and what we need to know. *Journal of Periodontal & Implant Science*, 46:136-151. PMID: 27382503

5. de Waal Y., Eijsbouts H., Winkel E., van Winkelhoff A. (2016) Microbial characteristics of peri-implantitis: a case-control study. *Journal of Periodontology*, Sep 26 [Epub ahead of print]. PMID: 27666672

6. Perez-Chaparro P., Duarte P., Shibli J. et al. (2016) The current weight of evidence of the microbiologic profile associated with peri-implantitis: a systematic review. *Journal of Periodontology*, 87:1295-1304. PMID: 27420109

7. Ogata Y., Nakayama Y., Tatsumi J. et al. (2016) Prevalence and risk factors for peri-implant diseases in Japanese adult dental patients. *Journal of Oral Science*, Oct 7 [Epub ahead of print]. PMID: 27725369

8. Lachmann S., Stehberger A., Axmann D., Weber H. (2013) The peri-implant health in patients attending an annual recall program. A clinical and microbiological study in 74 patients from the Tubingen Implant Registry. *Clinical Oral Implants Research*, 24:1300-1309. PMID: 22905716

9. Montevecchi M., Angelini F., Checchi V. et al. (2016) Microbiological distribution of six periodontal pathogens between untreated Italian and Dutch periodontal patients. *Oral Health & Preventive Dentistry*, 14:329-337. PMID: 26870849

10. Austin S., Bailey D., Chandu A. et al. (2015) Analysis of commonly reported medical conditions amongst patients receiving dental implant therapy in private practice. *Australian Dental Journal*, 60:343-352. PMID: 25330368

11. Lindhe J., Meyle J. (2008) Peri-implant diseases: Consensus Report of the Sixth European Workshop on Periodontology. *Journal of Clinical Periodontology*, 35:282-285. PMID: 18724855

12. Zitzmann N., Berglundh T. (2008) Definition and prevalence of peri-implant diseases. *Journal of Clinical Periodontol*

13. Gurgel B., Montenegro S., Dantas P. et al. (2016) Frequency of peri-implant diseases and associated factors. *Clinical Oral Implants Research*, Aug 24 [Epub ahead of print]. PMID: 27557997

14. Esposito M., Hirsch J., Lekholm U., Thomsen P. (2008) Biological factors contributing to failures of osseointegrated oral implants. (I). Success criteria and epidemiology. *European Journal of Oral Sciences*, 106:527-551. PMID: 9527353

15. Esposito M., Hirsch J., Lekholm U., Thomsen P. (2008a) Biological factors contributing to failures of osseointegrated oral implants. (II). Etiopathogenesis. *European Journal of Oral Sciences*, 106:721-764. PMID: 9672097

16. Alvarez-Camino J., Valmaseda-Castellon E., Gay-Escoda C. (2013) Immediate implants placed in fresh sockets associated to periapical infectious processes. A systemic review. *Medicina Oral, Patologia Oral y Cirugia Bucal*, 18:e780-e785. PMID: 23722139

17. Casap N., Zeltser C., Wexler A. et al. (2007) Immediate placement of dental implants into debrided infected dentoalveolar sockets. *Journal of Oral and Maxillofacial Surgery*, 65:384-392. PMID: 17307582

18. Lazzara R. (1989) Immediate implant placement into extraction sites: surgical and restorative advantages. *The International Journal of Periodontics & Restorative Dentistry*, 9:332-343. PMID: 2640210

19. Chen S., Wilson Jr. T., Hammerle C. (2004) Immediate or early placement of implants following tooth extraction: review of biologic basis, clinical procedures, and outcomes. *The International Journal of Oral & Maxillofacial Implants*, 19 Suppl:12-25. PMID: 15635942

20. Romanos G., Froum S., Hery C. et al. (2010) Survival rate of immediately vs delayed loaded implants: analysis of the current literature. *The Journal of Oral Implantology*, 36:315-324. PMID: 20735268

21. Konstantinidis I., Kotsakis G., Gerdes S., Walter M. (2015) Cross-sectional study on the prevalence and risk indicators of peri-implant diseases. *European Journal of Oral Implantology*, 8:75-88. PMID: 25738181

22. Marcantonio C., Nicoli L., Marcantonio E., Zandim-Barcelos D. (2015) Prevalence and possible risk factors of peri-implantitis: a concept review. *The Journal of Contemporary Dental Practice*, 16:750-757. PMID: 26522602

23. Derks J., Schaller D., Hakansson J. et al. (2016a) Peri-implantitis—onset and pattern of progression. *Journal of Clinical Periodontology*, 43:383-388. PMID: 26900869

24. Rokn A., Aslroosta H., Akbari S. et al. (2016) Prevalence of peri-implantitis in patients not participating in well-designed supportive periodontal treatments: a cross-sectional study. *Clinical Oral Implants Research*, Feb 26 [Epub ahead of print]. PMID: 26919480

25. Misch C., Perel M., Wang H. et al. (2008) Implant success, survival, and failure: The International Congress of Oral Implantologists (ICOI) Pisa Consensus Conference. *Implant Dentistry*, 17:5-15. PMID: 18332753

26. Benic G., Bernasconi M., Jung R., Hammerle C. (2016) Clinical and radiographic intra-subject comparison of implants placed with or without bone regeneration: 15-year results. *Journal of Clinical Periodontology*, Dec 15 [Epub ahead of print]. PMID: 27978603

27. Knofler W., Barth T., Graul R., Krampe D. (2016) Retrospective analysis of 10,000 implants from insertion up to 20 years—analysis of implantations using augmentative procedures. *International Journal of Implant Dentistry*, 2:25. PMID: 27915417

28. Marconcini S., Barone A., Gelpi F. et al. (2013) Immediate implant placement in infected areas: a case series. *Journal of Periodontology*, 84:196-202. PMID: 22509756

29. Barone A., Marconcini S., Giammarinaro E. et al. (2016) Clinical outcomes of implants placed in extraction sockets and immediately restored: a 7-year single-cohort prospective study. *Clinical Implant Dentistry and Related Research*, 18:1103-1112. PMID: 26888632

30. Chrcanovic B., Kisch J., Albrektsson T., Wennerberg A. (2016) Survival of dental implants placed in sites of previously failed implants. *Clinical Oral Implants Research*, Oct 14 [Epub ahead of print]. PMID: 27743398

31. Crespi R., Cappare P., Crespi G. et al. (2016) Immediate implant placement in sockets with asymptomatic apical periodontitis. *Clinical Implant Dentistry and Related Research*, Apr 28 [Epub ahead of print]. PMID: 27126371

32. Crespi R., Cappare P., Crespi G. et al. (2016a) Dental implants placed in periodontally infected sites in humans. *Clinical Implant Dentistry and Related Research*, May 16 [Epub ahead of print]. PMID: 27183325

33. Han C., Mangano F., Mortellaro C., Park K. (2016) Immediate loading of tapered implants placed in postextraction sockets and healed sites. *The Journal of Craniofacial Surgery*, 27:1220-1227. PMID: 27391493

34. Henningsen A., Smeets R., Wahidi A. et al. (2016) The feasibility of immediately loading dental implants in edentulous jaws. *Journal of Periodontal & Implant Science*, 46:234-243. PMID: 27588213

35. Srinivasan M., Meyer S., Mombelli A., Muller F. (2016) Dental implants in the elderly population: a systematic review and meta-analysis. *Clinical Oral Implants Research*, Jun 7 [Epub ahead of print]. PMID: 27273468

36. Zhou W., Want F., Monje A. et al. (2016) Feasibility of dental implant replacement in failed sites: a systematic review. *The International Journal of Oral & Maxillofacial Implants*, 31:535-545. PMID: 27183062

37. Pieralli S., Kohal R., Jung R. et al. (2017) Clinical outcomes of zirconia dental implants. *Journal of Dental Research*, 96:38-46. PMID: 27625355

38. Derks J., Schaller D., Hakansson J. et al. (2016) Effectiveness of implant therapy analyzed in a Swedish population: prevalence of peri-implantitis. *Journal of Dental Research*, 95:43-49. PMID: 26701919

39. Perka C., Haas N. (2011) Periprosthetic infection. [Article in German]. *Der Chirurg*, 82:218-226. PMID: 21340589

40. Bakathir A., Moos K., Ayoub A., Bagg J. (2009) Factors contributing to the spread of odontogenic infections: a prospective pilot study. *Sultan Qaboos University Medical Journal*, 9:296-304. PMID: 21509313

41. Hauser-Gerspach I., Vadaszan J., Deronjic I. et al. (2012) Influence of gaseous ozone in peri-implantitis: bactericidal efficacy and cellular response. An *in vitro* study using titanium and zirconia. *Clinical Oral Investigations*, 16:1049-1059. PMID: 21842144

42. Esposito M., Grusovin M., Worthington H. (2013) Interventions for replacing missing teeth: antibiotics at dental implant placement to prevent complications. *The Cochrane Database of Systematic Reviews*, 7:CD004152. PMID: 23904048

43. Romanos G. (2015) Current concepts in the use of lasers in periodontal and implant dentistry. *Journal of Indian Society of Periodontology*, 19:490-494. PMID: 26644712

44. Alshehri F. (2016) The role of lasers in the treatment of peri-implant diseases: a review. *The Saudi Dental Journal*, 28:103-108. PMID: 27656076

45. Pommer B., Haas R., Mailath-Pokorny G. et al. (2016) Periimplantitis treatment: long-term comparison of laser decontamination and implantoplasty surgery. *Implant Dentistry*, 25:646-649. PMID: 27504533

46. Salvi G., Cosgarea R., Sculean A. (2017) Prevalence and mechanisms of peri-implant diseases. *Journal of Dental Research*, 96:31-37. PMID: 27680028

Chapter 9

1. Levy T., Huggins H. (1996) Routine dental extractions routinely produce cavitations. *Journal of Advancement in Medicine*, 9:235-249.

2. Yoneda T., Hagino H., Sugimoto T. et al. (2016) Antiresorptive agent-related osteonecrosis of the jaw: position paper 2017 of the Japanese Allied Committee on osteonecrosis of the jaw. *Journal of Bone and Mineral Metabolism*, Dec 29 [Epub ahead of print]. PMID: 28035494

3. Vinitzky-Brener I., Ibanez-Mancera N., Aguilar-Rojas A., Alvarez-Jardon A. (2017) Knowledge of bisphosphonate-related osteonecrosis of the jaws among Mexican dentists. *Medicina Oral, Patologia Oral y Cirugia Bucal*, 22:e84-e87. PMID: 27918741

4. Black G. (1915) *A Work on Special Dental Pathology*, Chicago: Medico-Dental Publishing Co.

5. Bouquot J., Roberts A., Person P., Christian J. (1992) Neuralgia-inducing cavitational osteonecrosis (NICO). Osteomyelitis in 224 jawbone samples from patients with facial neuralgia. *Oral Medicine, Oral Surgery, and Oral Pathology*, 73:307-319. PMID: 1545963

6. Bouquot J., LaMarche M. (1999) Ischemic osteonecrosis under fixed partial denture pontics: radiographic and microscopic features in 38 patients with chronic pain. *The Journal of Prosthetic Dentistry*, 9922427

7. Gruppo R., Glueck C., McMahon R. et al. (1996) The pathophysiology of alveolar osteonecrosis of the jaw: anticardiolipin antibodies, thrombophilia, and hypofibrinolysis. *The Journal of Laboratory and Clinical Medicine*, 127:481-488. PMID: 8621985

8. Lechner J., von Baehr V. (2013) RANTES and fibroblast growth factor 2 in jawbone cavitations: triggers for systemic disease? *International Journal of General Medicine*, 6:277-290. PMID: 23637551

9. Tozum T., Demiralp B. (2003) Platelet-rich plasma: a promising innovation in dentistry. *Journal of the Canadian Dental Association*, 69:664. PMID: 14611717

10. Lacci K., Dardik A. (2010) Platelet-rich plasma: support for its use in wound healing. *Yale Journal of Biology and Medicine*, 83:1-9. PMID: 20351977

11. Dhurat R., Sukesh M. (2014) Principles and methods of preparation of platelet-rich plasma: a review and author's perspective. *Journal of Cutaneous and Aesthetic Surgery*, 7:189-197. PMID: 25722595

12. Jain N., Gulati M. (2016) Platelet-rich plasma: a healing virtuoso. *Blood Research*, 51:3-5. PMID: 27104183

13. Brown D. (2009) Complete edentulism prior to the age of 65 years is associated with all-cause mortality. *Journal of Public Health Dentistry*, 69:260-266. PMID: 19453862

14. Ando A., Tanno K., Ohsawa M. et al. (2014) Associations of number of teeth with risks for all-cause mortality and cause-specific mortality in middle-aged and elderly men in the northern part of Japan: the Iwate-KENCO study. *Community Dentistry and Oral Epidemiology*, 42:358-365. PMID: 24476489

15. Hirotomi T., Yoshihara A., Ogawa H., Miyazaki H. (2015) Number of teeth and 5-year mortality in an elderly population. *Community Dentistry and Oral Epidemiology*, 43:226-231. PMID: 25600364

16. Hu H., Lee Y., Lin S. et al. (2015) Association between tooth loss, body mass index, and all-cause mortality among elderly patients in Taiwan. *Medicine*, 94:e1543. PMID: 26426618

17. Joshy G., Arora M., Korda R. et al. (2016) Is poor oral health a risk marker for incident cardiovascular disease hospitalization and all-cause mortality? Findings from 172,630 participants from the prospective 45 and Up Study. *BMJ Open*, 6:e012386. PMID: 27577588

18. Vedin O., Hagstrom E., Budaj A. et al. (2016) Tooth loss is independently associated with poor outcomes in stable coronary heart disease. *European Journal of Preventive Cardiology*, 23:839-846. PMID: 26672609

19. Kebede T., Holtfreter B., Kocher T. et al. (2017) Association of periodontal destruction and diabetes with mortality. *Journal of Dental Research*, 96:56-63. PMID: 27680027

20. Polzer I., Schwahn C., Volzke H. et al. (2012) The association of tooth loss with all-cause and circulatory mortality. Is there a benefit of replaced teeth? A systematic review and meta-analysis. *Clinical Oral Investigations*, 16:333-351. PMID: 22086361

21. Holmlund A., Holm G., Lind L. (2010) Number of teeth as a predictor of cardiovascular mortality in a cohort of 7,674 subjects followed for 12 years. *Journal of Periodontology*, 81:870-876. PMID: 20350152

22. Watt R., Tsakos G., de Oliveira C., Hamer M. (2012) Tooth loss and cardiovascular disease mortality risk—results from the Scottish Health Survey. *PLoS One*, 7:e30797. PMID: 22363491

23. Schwahn C., Polzer I., Haring R. et al. (2013) Missing, unreplaced teeth and risk of all-cause and cardiovascular mortality. *International Journal of Cardiology*, 167:1430-1437. PMID: 22560949

24. Liljestrand J., Havulinna A., Paju S. et al. (2015) Missing teeth predict incident cardiovascular events, diabetes, and death. *Journal of Dental Research*, 94:1055-1062. PMID: 25991651

Chapter 10

1. Dlugaszewska J., Leszczynska M., Lenkowski M. et al. (2016) The pathophysiological role of bacterial biofilms in chronic sinusitis. *European Archives of Oto-Rhino-Laryngology*, 273:1989-1994. PMID: 26024693

2. Kennedy J., Borish L. (2013) Chronic sinusitis pathophysiology: the role of allergy. *American Journal of Rhinology & Allergy*, 27:367-371. PMID: 23601202

3. Lam K., Schleimer R., Kern R. (2015) The etiology and pathogenesis of chronic rhinosinusitis: a review of current hypotheses. *Current Allergy and Asthma Reports*, 15:41. PMID: 26143392

4. Min J, Tan B. (2015) Risk factors for chronic rhinosinusitis. *Current Opinion in Allergy and Clinical Immunology*, 15:1-13. PMID: 25479315

5. Taschieri S., Torretta S., Corbella S. et al. (2015) Pathophysiology of sinusitis of odontogenic origin. *Journal of Investigative and Clinical Dentistry*, Dec 14 [Epub ahead of print]. PMID: 26662929

6. McCarty J., David R., Lensing S. et al. (2016) Root cause analysis: an examination of odontogenic origins of acute maxillary sinusitis in both immunocompetent & immunocompromised patients. *Journal of Computer Assisted Tomography*, Oct 29 [Epub ahead of print]. PMID: 27798445

7. Kulacz R., Fishman G., Levine H. (2004) An unsuccessful sinus surgery caused by dental involvement within the floor of the maxillary sinus. *Operative Techniques in Otolaryngology—Head and Neck Surgery*, 15:2-3.

8. Akhlaghi F., Esmaeelinejad M., Safai P. (2015) Etiologies and treatments of odontogenic maxillary sinusitis: a systematic review. *Iranian Red Crescent Medical Journal*, 17:e25536. PMID: 26756016

9. Simuntis R., Kubilius R., Ryskiene S., Vaitkus S. (2015) Odontogenic maxillary sinusitis obscured by midfacial trauma. *Stomatogija*, 17:29-32. PMID: 26183855

10. Longhini A., Ferguson B. (2011) Clinical aspects of odontogenic maxillary sinusitis: a case series. *International Forum of Allergy & Rhinology*, 1:409-415. PMID: 22287475

11. Hoskison E., Daniel M., Rowson J., Jones N. (2012) Evidence of an increase in the incidence of odontogenic sinusitis over the last decade in the UK. *The Journal of Laryngology and Otology*, 126:43-46. PMID: 21933468

12. Patel N., Ferguson B. (2012) Odontogenic sinusitis: an ancient but under-appreciated cause of maxillary sinusitis. *Current Opinions in Otolaryngology & Head and Neck Surgery*, 20:24-28. PMID: 22157162

13. Shanbhag S., Karnik P., Sirke P., Shanbhag V. (2013) Association between periapical lesions and maxillary sinus mucosal thickening: a retrospective cone-beam computed tomographic study. *Journal of Endodontics*, 39:853-857. PMID: 23791251

14. Fadda G., Berrone M., Crosetti E., Succo G. (2016) Monolateral sinonasal complications of dental disease or treatment: when does endoscopic endonasal surgery require an intraoral approach? *Acta Otorhinolaryngologica Italica*, 36:300-309. PMID: 27734983

15. Bomeli S., Branstetter B., Ferguson B. (2009) Frequency of a dental source for acute maxillary sinusitis. *Laryngoscope*, 119:580-584. PMID: 19160401

16. Matsumoto Y., Ikeda T., Yokoi H., Kohno N. (2015) Association between odontogenic infections and unilateral sinus opacification. *Auris, Nasus, Larynx*, 42:288-293. PMID: 25638394

17. Pokorny A., Tataryn R. (2013) Clinical and radiologic findings in a case series of maxillary sinusitis of dental origin. *International Forum of Allergy & Rhinology*, 3:973-979. PMID: 24039196

18. Rosenthal P., Lundy K., Massoglia D. et al. (2016) Incidental paranasal sinusitis on routine brain magnetic resonance scans: association with atherosclerosis. *International Forum of Allergy & Rhinology*, 6:1253-1263. PMID: 27509266

19. Onisor-Gligor F., Lung T., Pintea B. et al. (2012) Maxillary odontogenic sinusitis, complicated with cerebral abscess—case report. *Chirurgia*, 107:256-259. PMID: 22712359

20. Coughlan C., Cerussi A., Kim J. et al. Near-infrared optical imaging for diagnosis of maxillary sinusitis. *Otolaryngology—Head and Neck Surgery*, 155:538-541. PMID: 27329417

21. Wang K., Nichols B., Poetker D., Loehrl T. (2015) Odontogenic sinusitis: a case series studying diagnosis and management. *International Forum of Allergy & Rhinology*, 5:597-601. PMID: 25732329

22. Troeltzsch M., Pache C., Troeltzsch M. et al. (2015) Etiology and clinical characteristics of symptomatic unilateral maxillary sinusitis: a review of 174 cases. *Journal of Cranio-Maxillo-Facial Surgery*, 43:1522-1599. PMID: 26319958

23. Jeong K., Kim S., Oh J., You J. (2016) Implants displaced into the maxillary sinus: a systematic review. *Implant Dentistry*, 25:547-551. PMID: 26974033

24. Kim S., Park J., Kim H. et al. (2016) Clinical features and treatment outcomes of dental implant-related paranasal sinusitis: a 2-year prospective observational study. *Clinical Oral Implants Research*, 27:e100-e104. PMID: 25675967

Chapter 12

1. Huggins H., Levy T. (1999) *Uninformed Consent. The hidden dangers in dental care.* Charlottesville, VA: Hampton Roads Publishing

2. Levy T. (2001) *Optimal Nutrition for Optimal Health.* New York, NY: Keats Publishing

3. Levy T. (2006) *Stop America's #1 Killer. Proof that the origin of all coronary artery disease is a clearly reversible arterial scurvy.* Henderson, NV: MedFox Publishing

4. Levy T. (2008) GSH, *Master Defender Against Disease, Toxins, and Aging.* Henderson, NV: LivOn Books

5. Levy T. (2011) *Primal Panacea.* Henderson, NV: MedFox Publishing

6. Levy T. (2013) *Death by Calcium. Proof of the toxic effects of dairy and calcium supplements.* Henderson, NV: MedFox Publishing

7. Kulacz R., Levy T. (2014) *The Toxic Tooth. How a root canal could be making you sick.* Henderson, NV: MedFox Publishing

8. Loria C., Klag M., Caulfield L., Whelton P. (2000) Vitamin C status and mortality in US adults. *The American Journal of Clinical Nutrition*, 72:139-145. PMID: 10871572

9. Khaw K., Bingham S., Welch A. et al. (2001) Relation between plasma ascorbic acid and mortality in men and women in EPIC-Norfolk prospective study: a prospective population study. European Prospective Investigation into Cancer and Nutrition. *Lancet*, 357:657-663. PMID: 11247548

10. Geleijnse J., Vermeer C., Grobbee D. et al. (2004) Dietary intake of menaquinone is associated with a reduced risk of coronary artery disease: the Rotterdam Study. *The Journal of Nutrition*, 134:3100-3105. PMID: 15514282

11. Ginde A., Scragg R., Schwartz R., Camargo Jr. C. (2009) Prospective study of serum 25-hydroxyvitamin D level, cardiovascular disease mortality, and all-cause mortality in older U.S. adults. *Journal of the American Geriatrics Society*, 57:1595-1603. PMID: 19549021

12. Semba R., Houston D., Bandinelli S. et al. (2010) Relationship of 25-hydroxyvitamin D with all-cause and cardiovascular disease mortality in older community-dwelling adults. *European Journal of Clinical Nutrition*, 64:203-209. PMID: 19953106

13. Reffelmann T, Ittermann T., Dorr M. et al. (2011) Low serum magnesium concentrations predict cardiovascular and all-cause mortality. *Atherosclerosis*, 219:280-284. PMID: 21703623

Chapter 13

1. Bocci V. (2004) Ozone as Janus: this controversial gas can be either toxic or medically useful. *Mediators of Inflammation*, 13:3-11. PMID: 15203558

2. Bocci V. (2011) *Ozone. A New Medical Drug*. Second Edition. New York, NY:Springer.

3. Bocci V., Luzzi E., Corradeschi F. et al. (1993) Studies on the biological effects of ozone: 4. Cytokine production and glutathione levels in human erythrocytes. *Journal of Biological Regulators and Homeostatic Agents*, 7:133-138. PMID: 8023701

4. Larini A., Bianchi L., Bocci V. (2003) The ozone tolerance: I) enhancement of antioxidant enzymes is ozone dose-dependent in Jurkat cells. *Free Radical Research*, 37:1163-1168. PMID: 14703728

5. Verdin E. (2016) NAD+ in aging, metabolism, and neurodegeneration. *Science*, 350:1208-1213. PMID: 26785480

6. Yamato M., Kawano K., Yamanaka Y. et al. (2016) TEMPOL increases NAD(+) and improves redox imbalance in obese mice. *Redox Biology*, 8:316-322. PMID: 26942863

7. Rilling S., Viebahn R. (1987) *The Use of Ozone in Medicine*, Second Revised Edition, First English Edition. Heidelberg:Haug.

8. Bocci V., Larini A., Micheli V. (2005) Restoration of normoxia by ozone therapy may control neoplastic growth: a review and a working hypothesis. *Journal of Alternative and Complementary Medicine*, 11:257-265. PMID: 15865491

9. Kucuksezer U., Zekiroglu E., Kasapoglu P. et al. (2014) A stimulatory role of ozone exposure on human natural killer cells. *Immunological Investigations*, 43:1-12. PMID: 24063543

10. Valacchi G., Bocci V. (2000) Studies on the biological effects of ozone: 11. Release of factors from human endothelial cells. *Mediators of Inflammation*, 9:271-276. PMID: 11213910

11. Bocci V. (1999) Biological and clinical effects of ozone. Has ozone therapy a future in medicine? *British Journal of Biomedical Science*, 56:270-279. PMID: 10795372

12. Nogales C., Ferrari P., Kantorovich E., Lage-Marques J. (2008) Ozone therapy in medicine and dentistry. *The Journal of Contemporary Dental Practice*, 9:75-84. PMID: 18473030

13. Saini R. (2011) Ozone therapy in dentistry: a strategic review. *Journal of Natural Science, Biology and Medicine*, 2:151-153. PMID: 22346227

14. Bocci V., Zanardi I., Borrelli E., Travagli V. (2012) Reliable and effective oxygen-ozone therapy at a crossroads with ozonated saline infusion and ozone rectal insufflation. *The Journal of Pharmacy and Pharmacology*, 64:482-489. PMID: 22420654

Appendix C

1. Levy T (2002) *Curing the Incurable. Vitamin C, Infectious Diseases, and Toxins.* Henderson, NV: MedFox Publishing

2. Klenner F (1971) Observations of the dose and administration of ascorbic acid when employed beyond the range of a vitamin in human pathology, *Journal of Applied Nutrition* 23:61-88.

3. Ayre S, Perez D, Perez D Jr. (1986) Insulin potentiation therapy: a new concept in the management of chronic degenerative disease, *Medical Hypotheses* 20:199-210. PMID: 3526099

4. Qutob S, Dixon S, Wilson J (1998) Insulin stimulates vitamin C recycling and ascorbate accumulation in osteoblastic cells, *Endocrinology* 139:51-56. PMID: 9421397

5. Rumsey S, Daruwala R, Al-Hasani H, et al. (2000) Dehydroascorbic acid transport by GLUT4 in Xenopus oocytes and isolated rat adipocytes, *The Journal of Biological Chemistry* 275:28246-28253. PMID: 10862609

6. Musselmann K, Kane B, Alexandrou B, Hassell J (2006) Stimulation of collagen synthesis by insulin and proteoglycan accumulation by ascorbate in bovine keratocytes in vitro, *Investigative Ophthalmology & Visual Science* 47:5260-5266. PMID: 17122111

7. Klenner F (1971) Observations of the dose and administration of ascorbic acid when employed beyond the range of a vitamin in human pathology, *Journal of Applied Nutrition* 23:61-88.

8. Cathcart R (1981) Vitamin C, titrating to bowel tolerance, anascorbemia, and acute induced scurvy, *Medical Hypotheses* 7:1359-1376. PMID: 7321921

9. Cathcart R (1985) Vitamin C: the nontoxic, nonrate-limited, antioxidant free radical scavenger, *Medical Hypotheses* 18:61-77. PMID: 4069036

10. Kurtz T, Morris R Jr. (1983) Dietary chloride as a determinant of "sodium-dependent" hypertension, *Science* 222:1139-1141. PMID: 6648527

11. Kurtz T, Al-Bander H, Morris R Jr. (1987) "Salt-sensitive" essential hypertension in men. Is the sodium ion alone important? *The New England Journal of Medicine* 317:1043-1048. PMID: 3309653

12. Pokorski M, Marczak M, Dymecka A, Suchocki P (2003) Ascorbyl palmitate as a carrier of ascorbate into neural tissues, *Journal of Biomedical Science* 10:193-198. PMID: 12595755

13. Pokorski M, Gonet B (2004) Capacity of ascorbyl palmitate to produce the ascorbyl radical *in vitro*: an electron spin resonance investigation, *Physiological Research* 53:311-316. PMID: 15209539

14. Pokorski M, Ramadan A, Marczak M (2004) Ascorbyl palmitate augments hypoxic respiratory response in the cat, *Journal of Biomedical Science* 11:465-471. PMID: 15153781

15. Ross D, Mendiratta S, Qu Z, et al. (1999) Ascorbate 6-palmitate protects human erythrocytes from oxidative damage, *Free Radical Biology & Medicine* 26:81-89. PMID: 9890643

16. Loyd D, Lynch S (2011) Lipid-soluble vitamin C palmitate and protection of human high-density lipoprotein from hypochlorite-mediated oxidation, *International Journal of Cardiology* 152:256-257. PMID: 21872949

17. Gosenca M, Bester-Rogac M, Gasperlin M (2013) Lecithin based lamellar liquid crystals as a physiologically acceptable dermal delivery system for ascorbyl palmitate, *European Journal of Pharmaceutical Sciences* May 3. [Epub ahead of print]. PMID: 23643736

18. Sawant R, Vaze O, Wang T, et al. (2012) Palmitoyl ascorbate liposomes and free ascorbic acid: comparison of anticancer therapeutic effects upon parenteral administration, *Pharmaceutical Research* 29:375-383. PMID: 21845505

19. Levy T (2002) *Curing the Incurable. Vitamin C, Infectious Diseases, and Toxins.* Henderson, NV: MedFox Publishing

20. Levy T (2011) *Primal Panacea.* Henderson, NV: MedFox Publishing

21. Padayatty S, Sun A, Chen Q, et al. (2010) Vitamin C: intravenous use by complementary and alternative medicine practitioners and adverse effects, *PLoS One* 5:e11414. PMID: 20628650

22. Rawat A, Vaidya B, Khatri K, et al. (2007) Targeted intracellular delivery of therapeutics: an overview, *Die Pharmazie* 62:643-658. PMID: 17944316

23. Yamada Y, Harashima H (2008) Mitochondrial drug delivery systems for macromolecule and their therapeutic application to mitochondrial diseases, *Advanced Drug Delivery Reviews* 60:1439-1462. PMID: 18655816

24. Goldenberg H, Schweinzer E (1994) Transport of vitamin C in animal and human cells, *Journal of Bioenergetics and Biomembranes* 26:359-367. PMID: 7844110

25. Liang W, Johnson D, Jarvis S (2001) Vitamin C transport systems of mamma-
    lian cells, *Molecular Membrane Biology* 18:87-95. PMID: 11396616

26. Welch R, Wang Y, Crossman A Jr. (1995) Accumulation of vitamin C (ascor-
    bate) and its oxidized metabolite dehydroascorbic acid occurs by separate
    mechanisms, *The Journal of Biological Chemistry* 270:12584-12592. PMID:
    7759506

27. Ling S, Magosso E, Khan N, et al. (2006) Enhanced oral bioavailability and
    intestinal lymphatic transport of a hydrophilic drug using liposomes, *Drug
    Development and Industrial Pharmacy* 32:335-345. PMID: 16556538

28. Lubin B, Shohet S, Nathan D (1972) Changes in fatty acid metabolism after
    erythrocyte peroxidation: stimulation of a membrane repair process, *The
    Journal of Clinical Investigation* 51:338-344. PMID: 5009118

29. Mastellone I, Polichetti E, Gres S, et al., (2000) Dietary soybean phospha-
    tidylcholines lower lipidemia: mechanisms at the levels of intestine, endo-
    thelial cell, and hepato-biliary axis, *The Journal of Nutritional Biochemistry*
    11:461-466. PMID: 11091102

30. Buang Y, Wang Y, Cha J, et al. (2005) Dietary phosphatidylcholine alleviates
    fatty liver induced by orotic acid, Nutrition 21:867-873. PMID: 15975496

31. Demirbilek S, Karaman A, Baykarabulut A, et al. (2006)
    Polyenylphosphatidylcholine pretreatment ameliorates ischemic acute renal
    injury in rats, *International Journal of Urology* 13:747-753. PMID: 16834655

32. Levy T (2002) *Curing the Incurable. Vitamin C, Infectious Diseases, and
    Toxins.* Henderson, NV: MedFox Publishing

33. Klenner F (1971) Observations of the dose and administration of ascorbic
    acid when employed beyond the range of a vitamin in human pathology,
    Journal of Applied Nutrition 23:61-88.

Index

side effect of bisphosphonate drugs 208

source of pathogen-related toxins 111

Cavitation Diagnosis/Treatment
bacterial culture examination 323
debridement 214, 222, 313, 321
diagnosis of 319
linked to
increased all-cause mortality 222
ozone treatments 222, 241, 251, 273, 280, 316, 317
surgery 316, 321, 322

Cerebrovascular Disease
linked to 68
oral pathogens 56, 57, 68
periodontitis 52, 68, 69

Chronic Obstructive Pulmonary Disease (COPD)
linked to periodontitis 70
prevalence of 40, 41
risk factor for periodontitis 70

COPD. *See under* **Pulmonary Disease (COPD)**

Copper
cause of increased oxidative stress 76, 108
deficiency impossible 108
found in multi-nutrient supplements 109, 311, 312
intracellular role 107
linked to
cancer 108, 109
development of atherosclerotic plaques 108
heart attack 108
increased all-cause mortality 109
toxic nutrient 100, 107, 109, 259, 265, 300
upregulates Fenton reaction 107

Crohn's Disease (Inflammatory Bowel Disease)
linked to
excess dietary iron 120
periodontitis 53, 72

D

Dementia. *See also* **Alzheimer's Disease**
linked to
oral infections 35
periodontitis 63
pathophysiological abnormalities 254
prevalence of 44, 48
treatment costs 48

Dental Implantitis Diagnosis/ Treatment
diagnosis 203
3D cone beam imaging 204
C-reactive protein levels 203, 204
X-ray 204
treatment 249
antibiotic therapy 204
guided bone regeneration 204
implantoplasty surgery 204
laser decontamination 204
ozone therapy 204, 277

Dental Implants
clinical impact 194, 196
description 193, 200
evaluating success vs failure 195, 196, 198, 201, 202
expense of 205
failure 203
infected (peri-implantitis) 194, 195
clinical impact 199, 239
infected sinuses 225, 231
mechanical failure of implant 197, 200
presence of periodontal pathogens 195
resorption of surrounding bone 195
similar to periodontitis 194, 195
prevalence of 194, 196, 197, 199
risk factors for 197
source of increased oxidative stress 112
toxicity of 171
infected (peri-implant mucositis) 194, 195
prevalence of 199

deficiency increases all-cause
mortality 95

foundational supplement 264

requires periodic testing of blood
levels 95, 237

supplement guidelines 311

the common "partner" of calcium
supplementation 101

toxicity from excess 95

increases all-cause mortality 95

Vitamin E 264

supplement guidelines 311

toxicity from excess in rare cases
95

Vitamin K

foundational supplement 264

safety 95

supplement guidelines 312

toxic level yet to be defined 96

Vitamins, Fat-Soluble. *See* **Vitamins
A, D, E, and K**

Vitamins, Water-Soluble.
See **Vitamins C and B**

X

X-ray *See also* **3D Cone Beam
Imaging**

as a diagnostic tool 234, 235, 236,
243, 244, 248, 261, 303, 305,
314, 315, 319

cannot be used as definitive reassurance that sinuses are normal
231

compared to 3D cone beam imaging
166, 168, 305

evidence of cavitations 207, 208

evidence of chronic apical periodontitis (CAP) 38, 39, 41, 74, 111,
145, 147, 152, 155, 157, 162,
164, 167, 168, 171, 172, 174,
180, 191, 241, 295

should never be ignored 161

intraoral

compared to 3D cone beam
imaging 167

compared to panoramic X-rays
167

of dental implants 201, 204

panoramic (full-mouth) 166, 167

radiolucency 145, 155, 157, 163,
164, 247

radio-opacity 145